ADHD RATING SCALE–5 FOR CHILDREN AND ADOLESCENTS

Also Available

ADHD in the Schools, Third Edition:
Assessment and Intervention Strategies
George J. DuPaul and Gary Stoner

Homework Success for Children with ADHD:
A Family–School Intervention Program
Thomas J. Power, James L. Karustis, and Dina F. Habboushe

Promoting Children's Health:
Integrating School, Family, and Community
Thomas J. Power, George J. DuPaul, Edward S. Shapiro, and Anne E. Kazak

Strategy Instruction
for Students with Learning Disabilities, Second Edition
Robert Reid, Torri Ortiz Lienemann, and Jessica L. Hagaman

Teacher's Guide to ADHD
Robert Reid and Joseph Johnson

ADHD RATING SCALE–5 for Children and Adolescents

Checklists, Norms, and Clinical Interpretation

George J. DuPaul
Thomas J. Power
Arthur D. Anastopoulos
Robert Reid

THE GUILFORD PRESS
New York London

Published by The Guilford Press
A Division of Guilford Publications, Inc.
370 Seventh Avenue, Suite 1200, New York, NY 10001
www.guilford.com

Printed in the United States of America

This book is printed on acid-free paper.

Last digit is print number: 9 8 7 6 5 4

Library of Congress Cataloging-in-Publication Data

DuPaul, George J., author.
ADHD rating scale–5 for children and adolescents : checklists, norms, and clinical interpretation / George J. DuPaul, Thomas J. Power, Arthur D. Anastopoulos, Robert Reid.
p. ; cm.
Preceded by ADHD rating scale–IV / George J. DuPaul . . . [et al.]. 1998.
Includes bibliographical references and index.
ISBN 978-1-4625-2487-7 (paperback : alk. paper)
I. Power, Thomas J., author. II. Anastopoulos, Arthur D., 1954– , author. III. Reid, Robert (Robert Charles), 1950– , author. IV. Title.
[DNLM: 1. Attention Deficit Disorder with Hyperactivity–diagnosis. 2. Adolescent. 3. Child. 4. Psychiatric Status Rating Scales. WS 350.8.A8]
RJ506.H9
618.92′8589–dc23

2015025998

About the Authors

George J. DuPaul, PhD, is Professor of School Psychology at Lehigh University. He is author or coauthor of numerous publications on the assessment and treatment of children, adolescents, and young adults with ADHD, including *ADHD in the Schools, Third Edition.*

Thomas J. Power, PhD, is Director of the Center for Management of ADHD at The Children's Hospital of Philadelphia and Professor of School Psychology in Pediatrics, Psychiatry, and Education at the University of Pennsylvania. He has published widely on the assessment and treatment of children and adolescents with ADHD.

Arthur D. Anastopoulos, PhD, is Professor in the Department of Human Development and Family Studies at the University of North Carolina at Greensboro, where he also directs the ADHD Clinic. He regularly presents his work at scientific meetings and has published widely on the assessment and treatment of children, adolescents, and young adults with ADHD.

Robert Reid, PhD, is Professor in the Department of Special Education and Communication Disorders at the University of Nebraska–Lincoln. His research interests center on treatment of attention-related problems and cognitive strategy instruction. He is coauthor of *Strategy Instruction for Students with Learning Disabilities, Second Edition.*

Preface

Attention-deficit/hyperactivity disorder (ADHD) is one of the most common behavior disorders of childhood. Mental health and school practitioners frequently face the challenge of assessing children and adolescents who might have ADHD. After the publication of the *Diagnostic and Statistical Manual of Mental Disorders,* fourth edition (DSM-IV; American Psychiatric Association, 1994), we set out to create a brief questionnaire (i.e., the ADHD Rating Scale–IV) that would allow clinicians to quickly determine the frequency and severity of ADHD symptoms. The ADHD Rating Scale–IV has been used in dozens of assessment and research studies since its publication in 1998. Furthermore, the scale is widely used by medical, mental health, and educational practitioners for a variety of activities including screening, diagnostic assessment, and evaluation of treatment outcome.

Subsequent to the publication of DSM-5 (American Psychiatric Association, 2013), we updated the content of the scale in two ways. First, consistent with wording changes in ADHD symptoms for assessment of adolescents and adults, we created adolescent versions of the parent and teacher ratings to include wording that was specific for this age group (i.e., symptoms are described in developmentally appropriate ways). Second, given the critical importance of functional impairment for assessing ADHD, two sets of impairment items were added to the scale, one set reflecting impairment due to inattention symptoms and the other set evaluating impairment due to hyperactive–impulsive symptoms. In addition to changes in content, we have collected extensive data from two normative samples (one for parent ratings and one for teacher ratings) that are representative of the U.S. population with respect to region, racial and ethnic background, and socioeconomic status. We also present information about the concurrent validity of the newly created scale. Finally, we have provided comprehensive data regarding the clinical utility of this scale for screening, diagnosis, and treatment evaluation purposes.

Of course, a project of this magnitude could not be completed without the support and assistance of many individuals. First, normative data collection was conducted through the GfK Knowledge Panel®. We are especially grateful to Carolyn Chu with GfK for her oversight of data collection and consistent support in providing us with detailed information regarding the data collection and analysis process. Second, the efforts of co-investigators Matthew Lambert and Marley Watkins were integral to the completion of this project, particularly with respect to statistical analyses and interpretation of the normative data. Additional co-investigators Matthew Gormley, Brittany Pollack, Kristina Puzino, and Tia Bassano provided valuable contributions in the collection, analysis, and interpretation of reliability and validity data. We would also like to thank Dr. Brenda Tracy and the teachers of Norris School District, in Norris, Nebraska, and Bethlehem Area School District in Bethlehem, Pennsylvania, for their help with reliability data. The assistance of Brittany Woods in the preparation of Chapter 6 was invaluable. Finally, we appreciate the willingness of the thousands of parents and teachers who completed the ADHD Rating Scale–5 as part of our development and validation of this scale.

Contents

CHAPTER 1

Introduction to the ADHD Rating Scales

Attention-deficit/hyperactivity disorder (ADHD) is a diagnostic category used to describe individuals who display developmentally inappropriate levels of inattention, impulsivity, and/or motor activity (American Psychiatric Association, 2013). Epidemiological studies have found that ADHD affects approximately 5.9–7.1% of children and adolescents (Willcutt, 2012). In the United States, parents report that around 11% of children have received an ADHD diagnosis from community practitioners (Visser et al., 2014). Given the prevalence, chronicity, and myriad difficulties associated with this disorder, it is important for clinicians to use psychometrically sound instruments when evaluating children and adolescents suspected of having ADHD.

Purpose of the Manual

The purpose of this manual is to describe the ADHD Rating Scale–5, Home Version, and the ADHD Rating Scale–5, School Version. With the permission of the American Psychiatric Association, both rating scales are based on the diagnostic criteria for ADHD as described in the fifth edition of the *Diagnostic and Statistical Manual of Mental Disorders* (DSM-5; American Psychiatric Association, 2013). Information is presented about the development and standardization of these scales, collection of normative data, factor structure, psychometric properties (i.e., reliability and validity), as well as the interpretive uses of these scales in clinical and school settings.

Background and Description of the ADHD Rating Scale–5

Over the past three decades, the diagnostic criteria for ADHD have undergone several changes that have significantly altered the clinical assessment of this disorder. Research over the last 30 years has consistently demonstrated that ADHD symptoms can be divided into two separate factors of inattention and hyperactivity–impulsivity (e.g., Bauermeister et al., 1995; DuPaul, Power, Anastopoulos, & Reid, 1998). Based, in part, on these findings, DSM-5 provides diagnostic criteria organized into two dimensions of inattention and hyperactivity–impulsivity, each of which consists of nine symptoms. Recent research has also demonstrated that there was a need for slightly different symptom descriptors for children and adolescents. In particular, symptom descriptions that are developmentally relevant for adolescents and adults were added to the DSM-5 criteria for ADHD. Thus the ADHD Rating Scale–5 has incorporated the DSM-5 changes by creating separate forms for children and adolescents, with the adolescent form providing developmentally relevant examples of problem behavior based on DSM-5 descriptions. Finally, recent research stressed that it is crucial that symptoms result in functional impairment in common home and/or school situations. In fact, the DSM-5 requires symptoms to be associated with impairment in at least one functional area (e.g., academic performance, social relationships) for an ADHD diagnosis to be warranted. For this reason, the ADHD Rating Scale–5 has incorporated two impairment scales keyed to the inattention and hyperactivity–impulsivity dimensions. This allows users to assess the extent to which ADHD-related problems adversely affect the home and/or school functioning of children and adolescents.

An evaluation of ADHD typically involves multiple components that may include diagnostic interviews with the child and his or her parents and teachers, behavior rating scales completed by parents and teachers, direct observations of school behavior, and clinic-based testing (Barkley, 2015; DuPaul & Stoner, 2014). Although many behavior questionnaires are available for use in such evaluations, very few of the currently available instruments specifically include items directly adapted from the DSM-5 criteria for ADHD. Thus our purpose in creating the ADHD Rating Scale–5 was to provide clinicians with a method to obtain parent and teacher ratings regarding the frequency of each of the symptoms of ADHD based on DSM-5 criteria.

Eighteen scale items were written to reflect DSM-5 criteria as closely as possible while maintaining brevity. The primary change made to each symptom was to omit the word "often" from the symptomatic description because respondents are asked to indicate the frequency of each symptom on a 4-point Likert scale ("never or rarely," "sometimes," "often," or "very often"). Adapted descriptions of ADHD symptoms, based on wording used in DSM-5, are included for the adolescent version. Parents are asked to determine symptomatic frequency that best describes the child's or adolescent's home behavior over the previous 6 months (in accordance with DSM-5 guidelines), and teachers rate the frequency that best describes the student's school behavior over the previous 6 months or since the beginning of the school year. English and Spanish versions of the ADHD Rating Scale–5, Home Version: Child and Home Version: Adolescent are presented in the

Appendix, as is the School Version of the ADHD Rating Scale–5 for children and adolescents (English only).

Administration and Scoring

All versions of the ADHD Rating Scale–5 are designed to be completed independently by a child's parent or teacher. The respondent is instructed to provide demographic information (i.e., name of child, age, grade, and name of respondent) and to circle the number for each item that best describes the child's or adolescent's home (or school) behavior over the previous 6 months (or since the beginning of the school year if the teacher has known the student for less than 6 months). If the respondent skips any item, he or she should be asked to provide a rating for this item. If the respondent indicates a lack of opportunity to observe the behavior and skips an item, then this item is not included in the scoring of the scale. If three or more items are omitted, the clinician should use extreme caution in interpreting the scale for screening, diagnostic, or treatment evaluation purposes.

The home and school versions of the ADHD Rating Scale–5 consist of two symptom subscales: Inattention (nine items) and Hyperactivity–Impulsivity (nine items). These subscales are empirically derived (see Chapter 2) and conform to the two symptomatic dimensions described in the DSM-5. Thus three symptom scores (Inattention, Hyperactivity–Impulsivity, and total) are derived from each version. The Inattention subscale raw score is computed by summing the item scores for Items 1–9. The Hyperactivity–Impulsivity subscale raw score is computed by summing the item scores for Items 10–18. The Total Scale raw score is obtained by adding the Inattention and Hyperactivity–Impulsivity subscale raw scores.

The ADHD Rating Scale–5 was designed to include items reflecting six domains of impairment that are common among children with ADHD. One domain assessed by the ADHD Rating Scale–5 is relationships with significant others (family members for the home version and teachers for the school version). A second domain is peer relationships, which are frequently impaired among children with ADHD (Barkley, 2015). A third domain is academic functioning, which is perhaps the most common impairment among children with ADHD (DuPaul & Stoner, 2014). A fourth domain is behavioral functioning; impairment due to disruptive behavior has been universally recognized and is extremely common among children with the hyperactive–impulsive and combined presentations of ADHD. A fifth domain is homework functioning, which is commonly impaired among children with ADHD and is associated with academic problems, emotional difficulties, and disruptive behavior (Power, Werba, Watkins, Angelucci, & Eiraldi, 2006). A sixth domain is self-esteem, which is often impaired among children with ADHD due to the disproportionate amount of punitive feedback these children receive from adults and peers (Barkley, 2015).

When using the ADHD Rating Scale–5, respondents complete each set of six impairment items twice, first after rating the inattention symptom items and again after rating the hyperactivity–impulsivity items. They are asked, "How much do the above behaviors cause problems for your child (this student)?" Items are rated on a 4-point scale (no, minor, moderate, severe problem).

Raw scores are converted to percentile scores by using the appropriate scoring profile (presented in the Appendix) based on the child's gender and age. The raw score for a particular gender, age, and scale is circled in the body of the profile. The corresponding percentile score is displayed in the extreme right- and left-hand columns of the profile. Figure 1.1 displays a sample profile for symptom scoring the ADHD Rating Scale–5, Home Version, for a 7-year-old boy. This boy's mother provided ratings resulting in the following raw scores and percentiles: Hyperactivity–Impulsivity = 17 (93rd percentile), Inattention = 15 (91st percentile), and Total = 32 (94th percentile). Note that when a raw score is associated with more than one percentile score, the clinician should report the *lowest* of the possible percentile scores. Figure 1.2 displays a sample profile for scoring impairments using the ADHD Rating Scale–5, Home Version, for a 7-year-old boy. Note that a child's score on each impairment dimension reflects the *higher* of the two ratings on items pertaining to symptom-related impairment for that dimension. For example, if the child received a rating of 1 for homework impairment related to inattention and a rating of 2 for homework impairment related to hyperactivity–impulsivity, the child's score on the homework impairment dimension would be a 2. In this case, the child received the following ratings from his mother: Family Relations = 0 (65th percentile), Peer Relations = 2 (98th percentile), Homework = 1 (90th percentile), Academics = 1 (90th percentile), Behavior = 3 (99.5th+ percentile), and Self-Esteem = 1 (95th percentile).

In Chapter 2, we describe the factor analyses used to derive the subscales of the ADHD Rating Scale–5. Descriptions of the normative samples, as well as gender, age, and ethnic differences in scale scores, are given in Chapter 3. The reliability and validity of various versions of the ADHD Rating Scale–5 are detailed in Chapter 4. Chapters 5 and 6 provide clinicians with guidelines for the interpretation and use of the scales for diagnostic and treatment evaluation purposes.

Child's name: Glenn Brown Date: June 9, 2015 Age: 7

%ile	HI 5–7	HI 8–10	HI 11–13	HI 14–17	IA 5–7	IA 8–10	IA 11–13	IA 14–17	Total 5–7	Total 8–10	Total 11–13	Total 14–17	%ile
99+	27	27	26	21	27	27	27	27	50	53	52	47	99+
99	24	26	22	16	25	27	27	26	45	49	47	39	99
98	19	20	19	15	23	25	27	25	41	44	43	37	98
97	18	20	18	13	22	21	25	21	38	38	38	34	97
96	17	19	17	12	21	20	22	20	38	36	36	30	96
95	17	18	15	10	18	17	21	19	35	35	34	27	95
94	17	17	14	9	17	16	21	18	32	33	31	26	94
93	17	16	13	9	17	16	19	18	31	31	30	25	93
92	16	16	12	9	16	16	18	17	29	30	28	25	92
91	15	15	11	8	15	15	18	16	27	29	26	22	91
90	15	14	10	8	14	14	17	16	27	28	25	21	90
89	13	13	10	7	14	12	16	15	26	25	24	20	89
88	13	11	9	7	12	12	15	14	25	24	23	19	88
87	12	10	9	6	11	12	15	13	24	22	22	18	87
86	12	10	9	5	11	11	15	12	22	21	22	18	86
85	10	9	9	5	10	11	14	11	20	19	21	17	85
84	10	9	9	5	10	11	13	11	20	19	21	16	84
80	9	8	7	4	9	9	12	10	18	17	19	14	80
75	8	7	6	3	9	9	10	9	16	14	17	11	75
50	5	3	2	1	5	4	6	4	10	8	8	5	50
25	2	1	0	0	2	2	1	1	4	3	2	2	25
10	0	0	0	0	0	0	0	0	0	1	0	0	10
1	0	0	0	0	0	0	0	0	0	0	0	0	1

FIGURE 1.1. Sample symptom scoring profile on the ADHD Rating Scale–5, Home Version, for a 7-year-old boy. HI, Hyperactivity–Impulsivity; IA, Inattention.

Child's name: *Glenn Brown* Date: *June 6, 2015* Age: *7*

%ile	Family Relations				Peer Relations				Homework				Academics				Behavior				Self-Esteem				%ile
	5–7	8–10	11–13	14–17	5–7	8–10	11–13	14–17	5–7	8–10	11–13	14–17	5–7	8–10	11–13	14–17	5–7	8–10	11–13	14–17	5–7	8–10	11–13	14–17	
99.5+	3	3	3	3	3	3	3	3	3	3	3	3	3	3	3	3	(3)	3	3	3	3	3	2-3	3	99.5+
99			2				2	2		2										2		2		2	99
98	2	2		2	(2)	2					2			2				2	2		2				98
95				1				1	2			2	2		2	2	2			1	(1)			1	95
93		1	1		1	1	1							1								1	1		93
90	1								(1)	1			(1)					1	1						90
85											1	1			1	1	1								85
80								0																	80
75							0												0	0	0	0		0	75
70		0		0	0	0			0				0	0				0					0		70
65	(0)		0														0								65
60										0					0	0									60
55											0	0													55
50																									50

FIGURE 1.2. Sample impairment scoring profile on the ADHD Rating Scale–5, Home Version, for a 7-year-old boy.

CHAPTER 2

Factor Analysis

As noted in the previous chapter, the diagnostic criteria for ADHD have undergone changes over the years due, in part, to variant conceptualizations of the dimensions underlying this disorder. During the 1960s and 1970s, ADHD was viewed as consisting of a single dimension of hyperactivity and inattention (American Psychiatric Association, 1968). As research began to highlight the importance of problems with inattention and impulsivity in this syndrome, a tripartite model was developed wherein children had to meet criteria in three separate dimensions: inattention, impulsivity, and hyperactivity (American Psychiatric Association, 1980). When empirical investigation did not support this tripartite model, the diagnostic criteria were reconceptualized in DSM-III-R as constituting a unitary dimension (American Psychiatric Association, 1987). In 1994, DSM-IV again reconceptualized the diagnostic criteria and returned to a model with two dimensions: one that reflected problems with attention, and a second that reflected problems with hyperactivity and impulsivity. DSM-IV also included a requirement for impaired functioning across two or more settings (e.g., home, work, school). The current DSM-5 (American Psychiatric Association, 2013) has maintained the two-dimensional structure of the DSM-IV but has slightly altered the wording for some items and has changed symptom thresholds in adolescents. The impairment criterion was maintained.

In this chapter, we provide two different factor analyses that were conducted for both versions of the ADHD Rating Scale–5. Because the home and school versions of the ADHD Rating Scale–5 are based on the DSM-5 criteria for this disorder, it is critical for these scales to conform to the bidimensional structure of the diagnostic criteria list. Confirmatory analyses provided specific information about the adequacy of the structural model presumed to underlie the two versions of the scale and the underlying construct validity of the two versions of this scale (DuPaul et al., 2015). In addition, we provide factor-analytic information on the newly added impairment scale (Power et al., 2015).

General Procedures

A Web-based survey that took approximately 5 minutes and 9 minutes (i.e., less than 5 minutes per student), for parents/guardians and teachers, respectively, was used to collect data. Each parent/guardian rated one child. Each teacher rated two randomly selected students. Parents and teachers did not rate the same children (i.e., parent and teacher ratings comprised separate samples). Respondents received small stipends (less than $5) for completing ratings. To minimize missing data, participants were systematically prompted to complete all fields. As a result, complete data sets were produced for > 99% of child ratings. All ratings were collected during April–May 2014.

Sample and Procedures: Factor Analyses of the Home Version

Participants

A total of 2,079 parents and guardians (1,131 female, 948 male) provided data for the ADHD Rating Scale–5, Home Version. Parents and guardians were predominantly white non-Hispanic (64.1%) and ranged in age from 20 to 77 years (M = 41.57; SD = 8.23). Most parents were married (79.7%), had at least high school education or greater (86.4%), and were employed (72.3%). Household income ranged from less than $5,000 (2.7%) to $175,000 or more (5.7%) with median income between $60,000 and $74,999 and mean income between $50,000 and $59,999. The parent sample was recruited from all regions of the United States and included households from both metropolitan (86.4%) and nonmetropolitan (13.6%) locations. English was spoken in most (89.4%) households. The children (N = 2,079; 1,037 males, 1,042 females) rated by the parents ranged in age from 5 to 17 years (M = 10.68; SD = 3.75). Children were from white non-Hispanic (53.9%), black non-Hispanic (13.1%), Asian non-Hispanic (5.7%), Hispanic (23.4%), and other (3.9%) backgrounds.

Procedures

Parents were recruited through GfK®, a national research firm. Parents were selected using address-based sampling (ABS) that allows probability-based sampling of addresses from the U.S. Postal Service's Delivery Sequence File. Individuals residing at randomly sampled addresses were invited to participate through a series of mailings (in English and Spanish); nonresponders were phoned when a telephone number could be matched to the sampled address. This resulted in a sample that was representative of the U.S. population in terms of child age/sex, race/ethnicity, family income, and geographic distribution. Household members who were randomly selected indicated their willingness to join the panel by returning a completed acceptance form in a postage-paid envelope, calling a toll-free hotline and speaking to a bilingual recruitment agent, or accessing a dedicated recruitment website. A total of 4,219 individuals were initially contacted to participate in the parent sample, with 2,708 (64.2%) completing ratings and 2,079 (76.8%) qualifying based on desired quotas for child demographics (i.e., age, gender, race, ethnicity). If multiple children between the ages of 5 and 17 were present in a given household, parents were asked to provide ratings for one randomly selected child such that the number of cases was balanced across gender and age range.

Sample and Procedures: Factor Analyses of the School Version

Participants

A total of 1,070 teachers (766 female, 304 male) provided ADHD symptom ratings for the ADHD Rating Scale–5, School Version. Each teacher rated two randomly selected students (one male, one female) on their class rosters (see "Procedures"). Teachers were predominantly white non-Hispanic (87.3%) and reported a mean of 17.88 years of teaching experience (SD = 10.7). The teacher sample was recruited from all regions of the United States and included general (83.3%) and special education (16.4%) teachers. The students (N = 2,140; 1,070 males, 1,070 females) rated by the teachers ranged in age from 5 to 17 years (M = 11.53; SD = 3.54) and attended kindergarten through 12th grade. Most students attended general education classrooms (83.2%) and were from white non-Hispanic (54.8%), black non-Hispanic (12.7%), Other non-Hispanic (7.0%), Hispanic (24%), or biracial non-Hispanic (1.5%) backgrounds.

Procedures

Teacher data were collected via two national research firms: GfK and e-Rewards®. Initially, 1,509 teachers contacted by GfK were assigned to complete ratings. Of these, 1,019 (67.5%) completed ratings, and of these 474 (46.5%) qualified on the basis of meeting targets for demographic variables (e.g., student grade, race/ethnicity, geographic distribution) based on census data. To obtain the desired sample size of 2,000 students, additional teachers were recruited through e-Rewards market research; e-Reward panelists are selected based on having a relationship with a business (e.g., Pizza Hut, Hertz, Macy's). A double opt-in is required; panelists must reply to the initial email invitation and then to a follow-up confirmation email. Potential panelists' physical addresses are then verified against postal records. All respondents are required to have a valid and unique email address. Respondents answer a profiling questionnaire when enrolling and provide information regarding employment status. The e-Rewards respondents indicated employment as a full-time, regularly employed (i.e., not substitute) teacher. A total of 12,610 teachers were invited to participate; 1,399 (11.1%) completed ratings, with 596 (42.6%)

qualified for inclusion on the basis of student demographics (i.e., child grade, race, ethnicity, and geographic region). To ensure equal gender representation, all teachers were asked to provide symptom ratings for one randomly selected boy and one randomly selected girl on their class roster. Each student selected was based on a randomly generated number provided in the instructions. Thus, for example, the teacher might be asked to select the seventh girl on the class roster. This procedure was used for both students rated. Secondary school teachers were instructed to provide ratings for one randomly selected male and one randomly selected female in a randomly selected class.

Confirmatory Factor Analyses of the Home and School Symptom Scales

The focus of the factor analysis was to examine the fit of the theoretical two-factor DSM model. Mplus v7.11 (Muthén & Muthén, 1998–2014) was used for confirmatory factor analysis (CFA) models. We compared the two-factor model fit with two alternative factor models: (1) a single factor model and (2) a three-factor model (with separate Inattention, Hyperactivity, and Impulsivity factors). Because items were measured on a 4-point Likert-type scale, we treated the ratings as ordinal rather than continuous indicators of the latent factors. We used weighted least squares with mean and variance adjustments (WLSMV; robust WLS) to estimate each model and the factors were scaled using a fixed mean and variance approach. Missing data for the CFA models were minimal ($< 0.01\%$) and excluded from the analysis by using a pairwise-present.

The comparative fit index (CFI; Bentler, 1990), Tucker-Lewis index (TLI), and the root mean square error of approximation (RMSEA; Steiger & Lind, 1980) at its 90% confidence interval were used to assess model fit. The CFI and TLI are comparative fit indices representing the degree of improvement over the worst-fitting model (Boomsma, 2000). Both indices are scaled from 0 to 1, with values closer to 1 indicating better fit. CFI and TLI values of 0.95 or greater were used to indicate an acceptably fitting model (Browne & Cudeck, 1993). RMSEA reflects the degree of model misfit and is reported on a scale of 0 to 1, with values closer to 0 indicating better fit, with values close to .06 balancing Type I and Type II error rates (Hu & Bentler, 1999). In addition to examining the point estimate, the 90% confidence interval was also used to evaluate misfit, with upper limits lower than .08 representing acceptable fit. The chi-square difference test ($\Delta\chi^2$) and CFI differences (ΔCFI) were computed to assess the fit nested models (e.g., the one-factor vs. the two-factor model). Difference in CFI less than .01 indicated that the fit of the two models being compared were statistically equivalent. All models were specified without correlated residual variances between items.

Results

Table 2.1 shows the results of the CFA for the Home and School versions. For both versions, the single-factor model did not exhibit acceptable fit. For both parent

TABLE 2.1. CFA Results for Parent and Teacher Symptom Ratings

	df	CFI	TLI	RMSEA (90% CI)	$\Delta\chi^2$ (*df*)
Home Version (parents)					
Single-factor model	135	0.925	0.915	0.122 (.119–.125)	–
Two-factor model	134	0.978	0.975	0.066 (.063–.069)	398.25 (1)*
Three-factor model	132	0.985	0.983	0.055 (.052–.058)	139.55 (2)*
School Version (teachers)					
Single-factor model	135	0.966	0.962	0.130 (.127–.133)	–
Two-factor model	134	0.989	0.988	0.074 (.071–.077)	438.30 (1)*
Three-factor model	132	0.992	0.991	0.063 (.060–.066)	164.56 (2)*

Note. From DuPaul, Reid, et al. (2015). Copyright 2015 by the American Psychological Association. Reprinted by permission.

*$p < .001$.

and teacher ratings, the two-factor model demonstrated acceptable fit (CFI ≥ .96, TLI ≥ .95, RMSEA close to .06), with the upper limit of the RMSEA confidence interval within the acceptable range. The two latent factors were highly correlated, .75 [95% CI = .73, .77] and .80 [.78, .82] for parent and teacher models, respectively, which is consistent with previous research (Burns, Boe, Walsh, Sommers-Flanagan, & Teegarden, 2001; Ullebø, Breivik, Gillberg, Lundervold, & Posserud, 2012). The three-factor model demonstrated a statistically significant improvement in fit over the two-factor model for the parent ($\Delta\chi^2_{(2)} = 139.55$, $p < .001$) and teacher ratings ($\Delta\chi = 164.56$, $p < .001$); however, the small ΔCFI (< .01) between the models indicates that the improvement in fit is not practically meaningful. In addition, interfactor correlations for the Hyperactivity and Impulsivity factors generally exceeded their reliability, suggesting that the two-factor solution should be preferred (Gorsuch, 1997). Figures 2.1 and 2.2 show the standardized factor loadings and the correlation between the latent factors for the Home (Figure 2.1) and School (Figure 2.2) two-factor models.

Summary and Conclusions

The results of the CFAs indicate that either a two- or a three-factor solution adequately represents the structure of this scale. Because the two-factor version conforms with the DSM-5 bidimensional diagnostic criteria, and the improvement for the three-factor model was not practically meaningful, we believe that the two-factor model best represents the scale. Items 1–9 can be totaled to derive an Inattention subscale score, and items 10–18 can be summed to obtain a Hyperactivity–Impulsivity subscale score. Clinicians can then use these two scale scores to determine a child's normative status with respect to the two domains of DSM-5 symptoms of ADHD. Separate scale scores may also aid in determining the ADHD presentation for a specific child or adolescent (see Chapters 3 and 5).

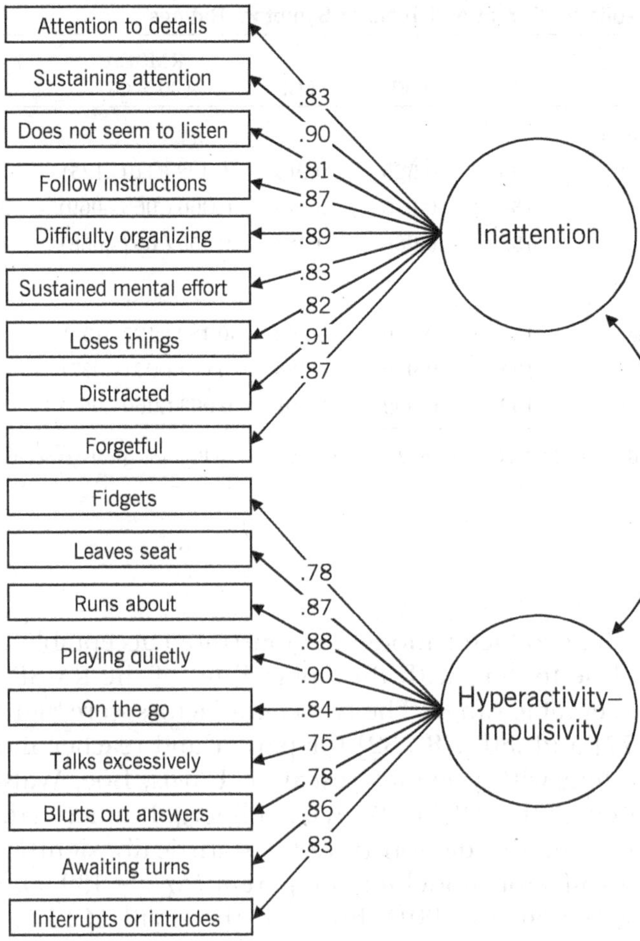

FIGURE 2.1. Two-factor model: parent report. From DuPaul, Reid, et al. (2015). Copyright 2015 by the American Psychological Association. Reprinted by permission.

Confirmatory Factor Analyses of the Home and School Impairment Scales

The samples used to assess the factor structure of the impairment scales for the Home and School ADHD Rating Scale–5 and the procedures to collect ratings were identical to those described previously. After respondents completed the Inattention items and the Hyperactivity–Impulsivity items, they were asked to complete six items assessing the extent to which problems with inattention (or hyperactivity–impulsivity) impaired functioning. Thus each respondent completed two impairment ratings for each child. Separate factor analyses were conducted for the Home and School versions.

Polychoric correlations and a weighted least squares estimator with mean- and variance-adjusted chi-square test statistics (WLSMV) were used to estimate factor models (DiStefano & Morgan, 2014) because the scale used ordinal items.

We tested three possible models: (1) the six Inattention impairment items and six Hyperactivity–Impulsivity impairment items would cluster into two correlated symptom-related factors (i.e., separate factors reflecting impairment for each symptom dimension); (2) the two items reflecting each of the domains of impairment (i.e., Teacher/Family Relationships, Peer Relationships, Homework, Academics, Behavior Problems, and Self-esteem) would form six separate factors; or (3) there would be one single factor composed of all 12 impairment items.

Model fit was evaluated with the CFI and the RMSEA. Criteria for adequate model fit were CFI ≥ .90 and RMSEA ≤ .08, whereas good model fit required CFI ≥ 0.95 and RMSEA ≤ 0.06 (Hu & Bentler, 1999). For a model to be considered superior, it had to exhibit adequate to good overall fit and display meaningfully better fit (ΔCFI > .01 and ΔRMSEA > .015) than alternative models (Cheung & Rensvold, 2002).

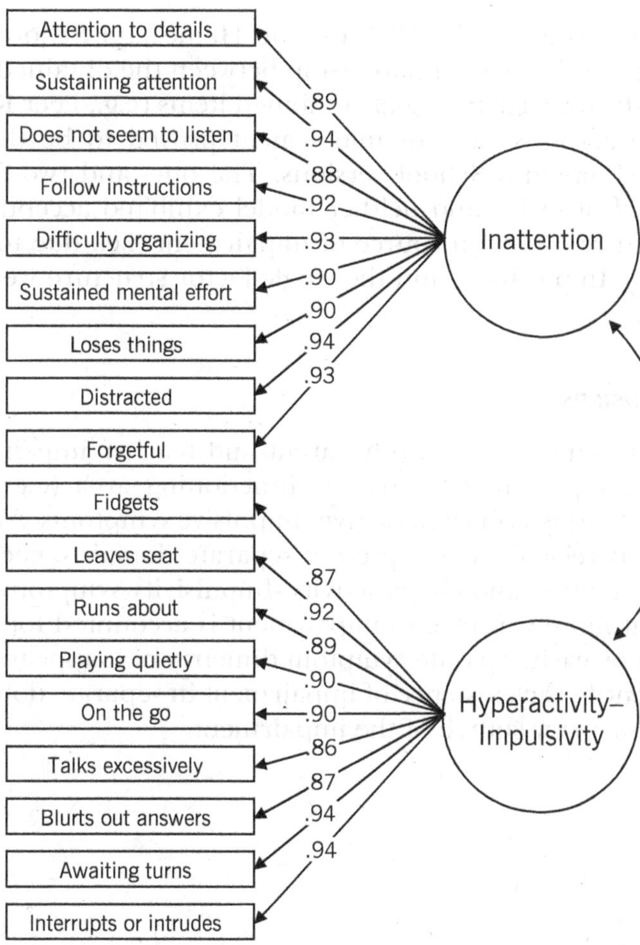

FIGURE 2.2. Two-factor model: teacher report. From DuPaul, Reid, et al. (2015). Copyright 2015 by the American Psychological Association. Reprinted by permission.

TABLE 2.2. CFA Results for Parent and Teacher Impairment Ratings

	χ^2	*df*	CFI	ΔCFI	RMSEA (90% CI)	ΔRMSEA
Home Version (parents)						
Single-factor model	2779.88	54	.959	–	.156 (.151–.161)	–
Two-factor model	2559.98	53	.962	.003	.151 (.146–.156)	.005
Six-factor model	240.46	39	.997	.035	.050 (.044–.056)	.101
Teachers						
Single-factor model	2900.58	54	.971	–	.157 (.152–.162)	–
Two-factor model	2707.72	53	.973	.002	.153 (.148–.158)	.004
Six-factor model	517.86	39	.995	.022	.076 (.070–.082)	.077

Note. From Power et al. (2015). Copyright 2015 Taylor and Francis Group. Reprinted by permission.

Results

Table 2.2 shows the results of the CFA for the Home and School impairment scale ratings. Figure 2.3 shows the relationship between the obtained factors. The model using the six-factor structure that combined items (e.g., Peer Relationships, Behavior Problems) across source of impairment proved to be the best-fitting structure for both Home and School versions. The one- and two-factor models were roughly equivalent in fit, and neither model exhibited acceptable fit. Both the two-factor structure based on source of impairment (i.e., due to Inattention, due to Hyperactivity–Impulsivity) and the single-factor structure were inferior to the six-factor model.

Summary and Conclusions

A six-factor structure emerged for both parent and teacher impairment ratings wherein each factor represented a specific functioning area (e.g., Homework) affected by both Inattention and Hyperactive–Impulsive symptoms. Although areas of impairment are correlated, they represent separate domains, each of which is affected by both Inattention and Hyperactivity–Impulsivity symptoms. The results further indicate that more variance in impairment is accounted for by ADHD as a whole rather than by each separate symptom dimension. It appears that respondents are able to identify the existence of impairment in separate domains but less able to identify the primary source of the impairment.

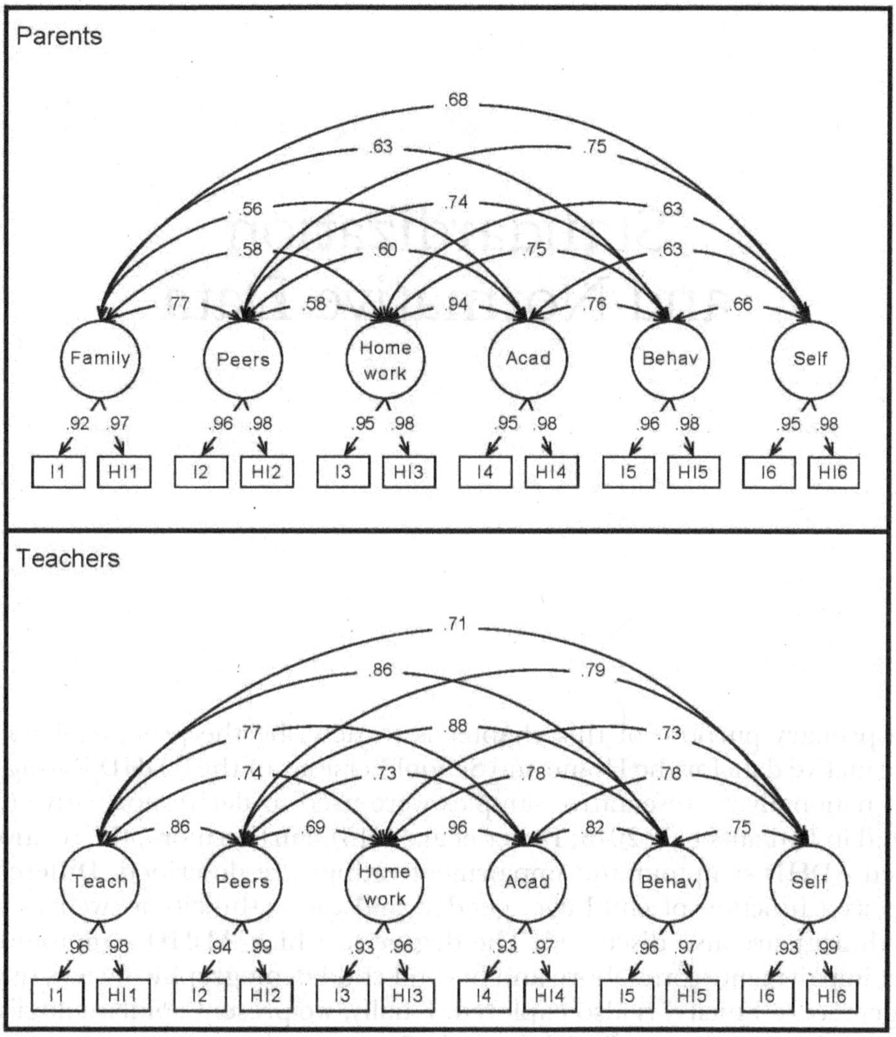

FIGURE 2.3. Six-factor structure of parent and teacher impairment items. Teach, Teacher Relations dimension; Acad, Academic dimension; Behav, Behavioral dimension; Self, Self-Esteem dimension. From Power et al. (2015). Copyright 2015 by Taylor and Francis Group. Reprinted by permission.

CHAPTER 3

Standardization and Normative Data

The primary purpose of this chapter is to describe the process of obtaining normative data for the Home and School Versions of the ADHD Rating Scale–5. Two nationally representative samples were used to derive normative data (as reported in DuPaul et al., 2015; Power et al., 2015). Furthermore, the relationships between ADHD symptom and impairment ratings are described. Differences in ratings as a function of child age, gender, and race/ethnicity as well as teacher race/ethnicity are also discussed. The degree to which ADHD symptom ratings predict impairment scores above and beyond child demographic factors (e.g., gender, age, race/ethnicity) is also explored. Finally, we present epidemiological data regarding the prevalence of ADHD clinical presentations in our normative samples.

Development of Normative Data: Samples and Procedures

ADHD Rating Scale–5, Home Version

Participants

As described in Chapter 2, the normative sample for the ADHD Rating Scale–5, Home Version was composed of 2,079 parents and guardians (1,131 female, 948 male) who completed ADHD symptom and impairment ratings for one of their children selected at random (see "Procedures"). Parents and guardians were predominantly white non-Hispanic (64.1%) and ranged in age from 20 to 77 years ($M = 41.57$; $SD = 8.23$). (See Table 3.1 for demographic characteristics of parent rating sample.) Most parents were married (79.7%), had at least high school education or greater (86.4%), and were employed (72.3%). Household income ranged from less than $5,000 (2.7%) to $175,000 or more (5.7%), with median income between

TABLE 3.1. Parent Ratings: Demographic Characteristics of Parents and Children

Parents (N = 2,079)		Children and adolescents (N = 2,079)	
Gender		Gender	
Male	948 (45.6%)	Male	1,062 (51.1%)
Female	1,131 (54.4%)	Female	1,017 (48.9%)
Age (years)		*M* age (years)	11.12 (3.80)
18–29	7.0%		
30–44	60.2%	Race/ethnicity	
45–59	31.2%	White, non-Hispanic	53.9%
60+	1.6%	Black, non-Hispanic	13.1%
		Other, non-Hispanic	5.9%
Race/ethnicity		Hispanic	23.4%
White, non-Hispanic	64.1%	Two or more races, non-Hispanic	3.5%
Black, non-Hispanic	13.1%		
Other, non-Hispanic	5.0%		
Hispanic	20.5%		
Two or more races, non-Hispanic	2.4%		
Education			
Less than high school	13.6%		
High school	25.3%		
Some college	26.6%		
Bachelor's degree or higher	34.5%		
Marital status			
Married	79.7%		
Widowed	0.4%		
Divorced	5.9%		
Separated	2.4%		
Never married	6.3%		
Living with partner	6.6%		
Household income			
Under $25,000	18.3%		
$25,000–$49,999	21.7%		
$50,000–$74,999	24.9%		
$75,000 and over	35.1%		
U.S. geographic region			
Northeast	16.6%		
Midwest	21.5%		
South	37.5%		
West	24.4%		

\$60,000 and \$74,999 and mean income between \$50,000 and \$59,999. The parent sample was recruited from all regions of the United States and included households from both metropolitan (86.4%) and nonmetropolitan (13.6%) locations. English was spoken in most (89.4%) households. The children (N = 2,079; 1,037 males, 1,042 females) rated by the parents ranged in age from 5 to 17 years (M = 10.68; SD = 3.75). Children were from white non-Hispanic (53.9%), black non-Hispanic (13.1%), Asian non-Hispanic (5.7%), Hispanic (23.4%), and other (3.9%) backgrounds.

Measures

Parents reported their gender, age, race, ethnicity, marital status, level of education, employment status, household income, and language spoken in the household. They also provided information about the children they rated including gender, age, race, and ethnicity. Parents reported the frequency with which each child displayed the 18 symptomatic behaviors of ADHD using one of four versions of the ADHD Rating Scale–5 depending on parent language (English or Spanish) or child's age (child or adolescent). With the permission of the American Psychiatric Association, items were created based on the wording of ADHD symptoms from DSM-5. Parents indicated the frequency of each symptomatic behavior on a 4-point Likert scale including 0 (never or rarely), 1 (sometimes), 2 (often), and 3 (very often). They were asked to select the number that best described their child's behavior over the previous 6 months. For adolescents ages 11 and older, additional wording (from DSM-5) was provided for some items to make these developmentally relevant. For example, the inattention item "has difficulty sustaining attention in tasks or play activities" was amended to include the following parenthetical text (e.g., "has difficulty remaining focused during lectures, conversations, or lengthy reading"). Parents whose primary language was Spanish (n = 236; 11.4%) completed a version of the ADHD Rating Scale–5 that included 18 symptom items using wording from the Spanish edition of DSM-5 (American Psychiatric Association, 2014). The translation process involved (1) initial translation into Spanish, (2) independent review by two specialists trained in language elements of diverse cultures, (3) collaboration between independent reviewers, and (4) involvement of a senior translator/researcher, if necessary, to resolve differences.

The ADHD Rating Scale–5 contains items reflecting six domains of impairment that are common among children with ADHD, including relationships with family members, peer relationships, academic functioning, behavioral functioning, homework performance, and self-esteem. Parent respondents completed a set of six impairment items twice, first after rating the inattention symptom items and again after rating the hyperactivity–impulsivity items. They were asked, "How much do the above behaviors cause problems for your child?" Items were rated on a 4-point scale (no, minor, moderate, severe problem).

Procedures

As described in Chapter 2, a large sample (N = 4,219) of parents were recruited through the GfK KnowledgePanel® to provide a sample of children and adolescents that was representative of the U.S. population in terms of race, ethnicity, geographic region, and family income (see Table 3.2). KnowledgePanel is a large national, probability-based panel that provides online research for measurement of public opinion, attitudes, and behavior. Panelists were selected using address-based sampling (ABS) that allows probability-based sampling of addresses from the U.S. Postal Service's Delivery Sequence File. Individuals residing at randomly sampled addresses were invited to join KnowledgePanel through a series of mailings (in English and Spanish); nonresponders were phoned when a telephone number could be matched to the sampled address. Household members who were randomly selected indicated their willingness to join the panel by returning a completed acceptance form in a postage-paid envelope, calling a toll-free hotline and speaking to a bilingual recruitment agent, or accessing a dedicated recruitment website. If more than one child between the ages of 5 and 17 was present in a given household, then parents were asked to provide ratings for one randomly selected

TABLE 3.2. Parent Ratings: Sample versus U.S. Census

Category	Percent sample	Percent Census[a]
Race/ethnicity		
White, non-Hispanic	53.9	53.55
Black, non-Hispanic	13.1	13.75
Hispanic	23.4	23.30
Other, non-Hispanic	5.7	5.85
Two or more races, non-Hispanic	3.9	3.55
Region		
Northeast	16.6	16.57
Midwest	21.7	21.50
South	37.5	37.61
West	24.4	24.32
Income level		
Under $25,000	18.3	18.63
$25,000–$49,000	21.7	21.71
$50,000–$74,999	24.9	17.65
$75,000 and over	35.1	42.01
Age (years)/sex		
5–7/boy	11.73	11.64
5–7/girl	11.15	11.13
8–10/boy	11.44	11.43
8–10/girl	10.87	11.09
11–13/boy	11.78	11.79
11–13/girl	11.21	11.17
14–17/boy	15.87	16.21
14–17/girl	15.39	15.54

Note. From DuPaul, Reid et al. (2015). Copyright 2015 by the American Psychological Association. Reprinted by permission.

[a]U.S. Population Benchmarks, March 2013, CPS Supplement Data.

child such that the number of cases was balanced across gender and age range. Of the 4,219 parents contacted to participate, 2,708 (64.2%) completed ratings and 2,079 (49.3%) qualified based on quotas for child demographic characteristics (e.g., grade, race/ethnicity, geographic region).

Parent ratings were completed through a Web-based survey that took approximately 5 minutes. Respondents received small stipends (less than $5) for completing ratings. If respondents left one or more items blank, they were prompted to complete missing items. Thus complete data sets were produced for > 99% of child ratings. All ratings were collected during April–May 2014.

ADHD Rating Scale–5, School Version

Participants

As described in Chapter 2, 1,070 teachers (766 female, 304 male) completed ADHD symptom and impairment ratings for two randomly selected students (one male, one female) on their class rosters (see "Procedures"). Teachers were predominantly white non-Hispanic (87.3%) and reported a mean of 17.88 years of

TABLE 3.3. Teacher Ratings: Demographic Characteristics of Teachers and Students

Teachers (*N* = 1,070)		Students (*N* = 2,140)	
Gender		Gender	
Male	304 (28%)	Male	1,070 (50%)
Female	766 (71.6%)	Female	1,070 (50%)
Age		*M* age	11.53 (3.54)
18–29	11.2%		
30–44	32.5%	Race/ethnicity	
45–59	41.8%	White, non-Hispanic	54.8%
60+	14.6%	Black, non-Hispanic	12.7%
		Other, non-Hispanic	7.0%
Race/ethnicity		Hispanic	24%
White, non-Hispanic	87.3%	Two or more races, non-Hispanic	1.5%
Black, non-Hispanic	3.1%		
Other, non-Hispanic	3.2%	Grade level	
Hispanic	5.0%	K–2	510 (23.8%)
Two or more races, non-Hispanic	1.5%	3–5	517 (24.2%)
		6–8	517 (24.2%)
M years of teaching experience	17.88 (10.7)	9–12	596 (27.9%)
U.S. geographic region		General education	1,782 (83.2%)
Northeast	23.2%	Special education	352 (16.4%)
Midwest	27.1%		
South	26.6%		
West	23.1%		
General education	891 (83.3%)		
Special education	176 (16.4%)		

teaching experience (*SD* = 10.7). (See Table 3.3 for demographic characteristics of teacher rating sample.) Teachers were recruited from all regions of the United States and included general (83.3%) and special education (16.4%) teachers. The students (*N* = 2,140; 1,070 males, 1,070 females) rated by the teachers ranged in age from 5 to 17 years (*M* = 11.53; *SD* = 3.54) and attended kindergarten through 12th grade. Most students attended general education classrooms (83.2%) and were from white non-Hispanic (54.8%), black non-Hispanic (12.7%), other non-Hispanic (7.0%), Hispanic (24%), or biracial non-Hispanic (1.5%) backgrounds.

Measures

Teachers reported their gender, age, race, ethnicity, years of teaching experience, and primary teaching assignment (i.e., general education or special education). They also provided information about the students they rated including gender, age, race, ethnicity, grade, and primary classroom placement (i.e., general education or special education). Teachers reported the frequency with which each student displayed the 18 symptomatic behaviors of ADHD using either the Child or Adolescent iteration of the ADHD Rating Scale–5, School Version based on the student's age (i.e., Adolescent version completed for students in grades 6–12). As was the case for parents, teachers indicated the frequency of each behavior over the past 6 months or since the beginning of the school year on a 4-point Likert scale including 0 (never or rarely), 1 (sometimes), 2 (often), and 3 (very often).

As was the case for parents, teachers rated student functioning across six domains including relationships with teachers, peer relationships, academic functioning, behavioral functioning, homework performance, and self-esteem. Teacher respondents completed a set of six impairment items twice, first after rating the inattention symptom items and again after rating the hyperactivity–impulsivity items. They were asked, "How much do the above behaviors cause problems for this student?" Items were rated on a 4-point scale (no, minor, moderate, severe problem).

Procedures

As described in Chapter 2, teacher data were collected via two national research firms: GfK Knowledge Panel and e-Rewards. Initially, 1,509 teachers on the KnowledgePanel® were contacted and 1,019 (67.5%) completed ratings. To obtain the desired sample size of 2,000 students, 12,610 additional teachers were recruited through e-Rewards market research; e-Reward panelists are selected based on having a relationship with a business (e.g., Pizza Hut, Hertz, Macy's). A double opt-in is required; panelists must reply to the initial email invitation and then to a follow-up confirmation email. Potential panelists' physical addresses are then verified against postal records. All respondents are required to have a valid and unique email address. Respondents answer a profiling questionnaire when enrolling and provide information regarding employment status. The e-Rewards respondents indicated employment as a full-time, regularly employed (i.e., not substitute) teacher. A total of 1,399 teachers (11.1% return rate) from the e-Rewards contact group completed ratings with 596 qualified based on quotas for child demographic characteristics (e.g., grade, race/ethnicity, geographic distribution). To ensure equal child gender representation, all teachers were asked to provide symptom ratings for one randomly selected boy and one randomly selected girl on their class roster. Each student selected was based on a randomly generated number provided in the instructions. Thus, for example, the teacher might be asked to select the seventh girl on the class roster. This procedure was used for both students rated. Secondary school teachers were instructed to provide ratings for one randomly selected male and one randomly selected female in a randomly selected class. Furthermore, the sample was recruited such that the number of cases was balanced across age and grade range and was representative of the U.S. child population in terms of race/ethnicity, geographic region, and age/sex (see Table 3.4).

Teacher ratings were completed through a Web-based survey that took approximately 9 minutes (i.e., less than 5 minutes per student). Respondents received small stipends (less than $5) for completing ratings. If respondents left one or more items blank, they were prompted to complete missing items. Thus complete data sets were produced for > 99% of child ratings. All ratings were collected during April–May 2014.

TABLE 3.4. Teacher Ratings: Sample versus U.S. Census

Category	Percent sample	Percent Census[a]
Race/ethnicity		
White, non-Hispanic	54.8	53.55
Black, non-Hispanic	12.7	13.75
Hispanic	24.0	23.30
Other, non-Hispanic	7.0	5.85
Two or more races, non-Hispanic	1.5	3.55
Region		
Northeast	23.2	16.81
Midwest	27.1	21.68
South	26.6	37.53
West	23.1	23.97
Age (years)/sex		
5–7/boy	11.1	11.64
5–7/girl	10.6	11.13
8–10/boy	11.8	11.43
8–10/girl	11.4	11.09
11–13/boy	12.3	11.79
11–13/girl	11.5	11.17
14–17/boy	15.9	16.21
14–17/girl	15.1	15.54

Note. From DuPaul, Reid, et al. (2015). Copyright 2015 by the American Psychological Association. Reprinted by permission.

[a]U.S. Population Benchmarks. March 2013. CPS Supplement Data.

Development of Normative Data: Results

Normative data for symptom ratings on the ADHD Rating Scale–5 are reported by age and gender for three scores: Inattention (IA), Hyperactivity–Impulsivity (HI), and total. Scores for IA and HI were calculated by summing item responses for the nine inattention and nine hyperactivity–impulsivity items, respectively. These two subscales reflect DSM-5 conceptualization of two domains for ADHD symptoms, and this structure has been confirmed empirically through factor analyses (see Chapter 2). Total score was calculated by summing responses for all 18 symptom items.

ADHD Rating Scale–5, Home Version

Normative data were computed separately for weighted parent ratings and presented for eight gender × age (5–7, 8–10, 11–13, 14–17 years) groups. Table 3.5 provides the means, standard deviations, and percentile scores for the IA, HI, and total scores for parent ratings. Four cutoff points are presented: 80th, 90th, 93rd, and 98th percentiles. These cutoff points can be used for screening risk (80th and 90th percentiles) and identification purposes (93rd and 98th percentiles) (Power, Doherty, et al., 1998; see Chapter 5). Although racial/ethnic differences in parent ratings were obtained (as described later in this chapter), normative data were not presented by race or ethnic group because there were insufficient numbers of participants for normative data to be displayed by gender, age, and racial/ethnic group.

Based on the findings from the confirmatory factor analyses (see Chapter 2) for the impairment items indicating that the optimal model had six factors, each consisting of the two items pertaining to impairment due to IA and HI corresponding with the six areas of impairment assessed, normative data are presented for each impairment factor. Scores for each impairment factor were created by selecting the higher of the two ratings on each factor. Frequency distributions for parent ratings on each impairment dimension as a function of age and gender are presented in Table 3.6. Most children had no or minor impairment problems, resulting in positively skewed distributions. Parent ratings indicated that 19.5% of the sample displayed moderate to severe problems on at least one impairment dimension (Table 3.6).

ADHD Rating Scale–5, School Version

Normative data were computed separately for weighted teacher ratings and presented for eight gender × age (5–7, 8–10, 11–13, 14–17 years) groups. Table 3.7 provides the means, standard deviations, and percentile scores for the IA, HI, and total scores for teacher ratings. Four cutoff points are presented: 80th, 90th, 93rd, and 98th percentiles. These cutoff points can be used for screening risk (80th and 90th percentiles) and identification purposes (93rd and 98th percentiles) (Power, Doherty, et al., 1998; see Chapter 5). Although racial/ethnic differences in teacher ratings were obtained (as described later in this chapter), normative data were

TABLE 3.5. Normative Data for Parent Ratings

		Inattention						Hyperactivity–Impulsivity						Total Score					
				Percentile						Percentile						Percentile			
Age	*n*	*M*	*SD*	80th	90th	93rd	98th	*M*	*SD*	80th	90th	93rd	98th	*M*	*SD*	80th	90th	93rd	98th
Males																			
5–7	244	6.14	5.79	9.0	15.0	17.0	23.0	5.78	5.35	9.0	15.0	17.0	18.9	11.92	10.31	18.0	27.0	31.0	40.0
8–10	238	5.74	5.40	9.0	12.0	16.0	21.4	4.48	5.58	8.0	13.0	16.0	20.0	10.21	10.20	16.0	25.1	30.0	42.4
11–13	245	6.41	6.13	11.0	15.0	17.0	25.1	3.63	4.73	7.0	10.0	11.5	19.0	10.05	9.82	18.0	23.0	25.5	38.0
14–17	331	5.42	5.93	9.0	14.1	18.0	21.1	2.33	3.52	4.0	8.0	9.0	13.8	7.74	8.73	13.0	20.0	25.0	36.0
Females																			
5–7	232	4.62	5.22	8.0	12.0	13.0	20.8	4.24	4.98	7.0	11.0	13.0	19.7	8.84	9.42	15.0	20.8	24.5	42.3
8–10	226	4.79	5.24	9.0	12.0	13.9	20.7	3.38	4.23	6.0	8.0	9.0	16.9	8.17	8.65	14.0	18.0	20.5	36.0
11–13	233	4.65	5.26	9.0	12.1	13.5	20.0	2.80	4.02	5.0	8.0	11.0	15.0	7.45	8.28	13.0	20.0	23.0	33.2
14–17	320	5.28	5.85	9.8	14.0	17.0	20.7	2.28	3.60	4.0	7.0	8.0	15.2	7.56	8.78	14.0	20.0	22.7	36.0

Note. From DuPaul, Reid, et al. (2015). Copyright 2015 by the American Psychological Association. Reprinted by permission.

TABLE 3.6. Percent Distribution of Parent-Rated Impairment Dimension Scores for Total Sample, for Males and Females, and for Age Groups

			Gender		Age group (years)			
Impairment	Score	Total	Male	Female	5–7	8–10	11–13	14–18
Family Relations	0—None	66.4	67.0	65.9	67.9	69.2	65.5	63.8
	1—Minor	25.0	25.4	24.5	24.4	24.3	25.5	25.7
	2—Moderate	6.9	5.9	7.9	6.1	5.2	7.9	7.8
	3—Severe	1.7	1.7	1.7	1.7	1.3	1.0	2.6
Peer Relations	0—None	74.3	73.8	74.8	74.1	72.7	75.1	75.1
	1—Minor	19.4	19.3	19.6	20.6	21.5	18.6	17.5
	2—Moderate	5.0	5.6	4.5	4.4	4.3	5.2	5.8
	3—Severe	1.2	1.3	1.1	0.8	1.5	1.0	1.5
Homework	0—None	64.9	59.1	70.9	73.7	66.6	63.7	58.3
	1—Minor	24.6	27.9	21.1	19.1	26.7	23.9	27.5
	2—Moderate	7.8	9.4	6.3	4.6	5.6	9.9	10.3
	3—Severe	2.6	3.6	1.6	2.5	1.1	2.5	3.8
Academics	0—None	69.3	64.4	74.4	77.7	71.6	66.5	63.6
	1—Minor	20.5	23.7	17.2	14.9	21.3	22.0	22.9
	2—Moderate	7.1	7.9	6.2	4.6	5.0	8.4	9.7
	3—Severe	3.1	3.9	2.2	2.7	2.2	3.1	3.8
Behavior	0—None	76.8	72.4	81.4	71.8	76.1	77.8	80.3
	1—Minor	17.0	19.8	14.1	19.8	17.8	14.7	16.2
	2—Moderate	4.2	5.3	3.1	5.9	4.3	5.5	1.8
	3—Severe	2.0	2.6	1.4	2.5	1.7	2.1	1.7
Self-Esteem	0—None	73.0	74.3	71.6	79.4	74.6	69.2	70.0
	1—Minor	20.7	19.1	22.4	16.8	19.1	22.6	23.2
	2—Moderate	5.0	5.5	4.5	2.5	5.8	6.9	4.8
	3—Severe	1.3	1.0	1.6	1.3	0.4	1.3	2.0

Note. Scores on each impairment factor were created by selecting the higher score on the two items of the factor (i.e., impairment related to Inattention and impairment related to Hyperactivity-Impulsivity). From Power et al. (2015). Copyright 2015 by Taylor and Francis Group. Reprinted by permission.

not presented by race or ethnic group because there were insufficient numbers of participants for normative data to be displayed by gender, age, and racial/ethnic group.

As was the case for parent ratings, confirmatory factor analyses (see Chapter 2) for the teacher-rated impairment items indicated that the optimal model had six factors, each consisting of the two items pertaining to impairment due to IA and HI corresponding with the six areas of impairment assessed. Scores for each impairment factor were created by selecting the higher of the two ratings on each factor. Frequency distributions for teacher ratings on each impairment dimension as a function of age and gender are presented in Table 3.8. Most children had no or minor impairment problems, resulting in positively skewed distributions. For teachers, 36% of the sample was identified as showing moderate to severe problems on at least one impairment dimension. In general, teachers provided higher

TABLE 3.7. Normative Data for Teacher Ratings

Age (years)	*n*	Inattention						Hyperactivity–Impulsivity						Total score					
				Percentile						Percentile						Percentile			
		M	*SD*	80th	90th	93rd	98th	*M*	*SD*	80th	90th	93rd	98th	*M*	*SD*	80th	90th	93rd	98th
Males																			
5–7	238	9.03	7.87	16.8	22.0	23.5	26.0	7.10	7.02	14.0	18.0	18.2	26.0	16.12	13.42	29.0	36.6	39.7	47.9
8–10	253	9.00	8.20	17.0	20.8	24.0	27.0	6.78	7.22	14.0	17.0	19.0	25.2	15.78	14.57	30.0	35.8	39.1	52.0
11–13	264	7.73	7.69	14.0	20.0	23.0	26.0	4.47	5.90	9.0	15.0	16.0	20.9	12.20	12.47	22.0	32.0	35.4	45.6
14–17	341	7.09	6.88	13.0	17.0	20.0	27.0	3.77	5.45	8.0	12.0	14.0	22.3	10.86	11.33	20.0	25.1	29.1	43.2
Females																			
5–7	228	6.09	6.93	13.0	17.0	18.0	23.0	4.84	6.11	9.0	14.0	17.0	22.0	10.93	12.29	23.3	30.0	33.0	42.1
8–10	244	5.33	6.54	10.0	17.0	18.0	23.9	3.06	4.71	6.0	11.0	13.0	16.9	8.39	10.43	17.0	24.0	28.6	39.2
11–13	247	5.63	6.85	10.0	17.0	18.3	25.0	2.68	4.24	5.0	9.0	9.7	15.0	8.31	9.98	17.0	24.0	27.0	33.1
14–17	324	3.45	4.94	7.5	10.0	11.1	18.0	1.53	3.17	2.0	5.0	7.2	12.0	4.99	7.36	9.0	14.0	18.2	28.0

Note. From DuPaul, Reid, et al. (2015). Copyright 2015 by the American Psychological Association. Reprinted by permission.

TABLE 3.8. Percent Distribution of Teacher-Rated Impairment Dimension Scores for Total Sample, for Males and Females, and for Age Groups

			Gender		Age group (years)			
Impairment	Score	Total	Male	Female	5–7	8–10	11–13	14–18
Teacher Relations	0–None	69.6	62.5	77.1	67.5	65.6	71.2	72.9
	1–Minor	19.9	24.0	15.5	21.4	22.9	18.8	17.3
	2–Moderate	9.0	11.4	6.5	9.4	10.1	8.2	8.6
	3–Severe	1.5	2.1	0.9	1.7	1.4	1.8	1.2
Peer Relations	0–None	63.0	57.3	69.0	51.3	56.2	67.3	72.8
	1–Minor	24.8	27.1	22.4	31.3	28.3	21.1	20.4
	2–Moderate	10.0	12.9	7.0	15.5	12.2	8.6	5.6
	3–Severe	2.2	2.7	1.6	1.9	3.2	2.9	1.2
Homework	0–None	49.3	41.8	57.2	49.7	50.2	45.2	51.4
	1–Minor	26.6	28.0	25.1	28.0	23.3	29.2	26.3
	2–Moderate	15.9	18.7	12.8	16.6	16.7	15.3	15.8
	3–Severe	8.2	11.5	4.8	5.8	9.8	10.4	8.2
Academics	0–None	49.6	42.0	57.6	48.2	47.5	50.8	51.5
	1–Minor	23.4	25.4	21.2	26.1	18.1	22.5	26.0
	2–Moderate	17.3	20.3	14.3	15.4	21.5	16.3	16.2
	3–Severe	9.7	12.4	6.9	10.3	12.9	10.4	6.3
Behavior	0–None	58.3	47.7	69.4	48.3	52.6	59.0	69.0
	1–Minor	21.9	25.3	18.4	24.0	21.4	25.8	17.9
	2–Moderate	14.2	19.2	8.9	19.5	18.1	10.7	9.9
	3–Severe	5.6	7.8	3.3	8.2	7.9	4.5	3.2
Self-Esteem	0–None	65.0	60.1	70.0	59.0	59.8	66.3	71.8
	1–Minor	22.8	24.8	20.6	25.8	25.1	22.1	19.4
	2–Moderate	9.6	12.2	7.0	11.4	11.8	9.8	6.8
	3–Severe	2.6	2.8	2.4	3.9	3.2	1.8	2.1

Note. Scores on each impairment factor were created by selecting the higher score on the two items of the factor (i.e., impairment related to Inattention and impairment related to Hyperactivity–Impulsivity). From Power et al. (2015). Copyright 2015 by Taylor and Francis Group. Reprinted by permission.

impairment ratings than parents. As shown in Table 3.9, 92.7% of the sample rated by parents displayed 0–2 total impairments; for teachers, this range increased, with 0–4 impairments accounting for a comparable percentage (92.6%) of the sample.

Relationships between ADHD Symptom and Impairment Ratings

The relationships between impairment ratings and IA, HI, and total symptom scores were quantified by the Spearman correlations that are presented in Table 3.10. Both parents and teachers reported stronger relationships between

TABLE 3.9. Frequency and Percentage of Impairments as Rated by Parents and Teachers

Number of impairments	Parents		Teachers	
	Percent	Cumulative	Percent	Cumulative
0	80.5	80.5	64.0	64.0
1	7.1	87.6	8.6	72.6
2	5.1	92.7	7.9	80.5
3	2.7	95.4	6.9	87.4
4	1.8	97.2	5.2	92.6
5	1.4	98.6	4.4	97.0
6	1.4	100	3.0	100

Note. An impairment was recorded as present if the informant rated the item as a moderate or severe problem; an impairment was recorded as absent if the informant rated the item as no or a mild problem. The "or" rule was applied if there was a discrepancy in ratings of the two items on the impairment dimension; the higher of the two ratings was determined to be the child's score. From Power et al. (2015). Copyright 2015 by Taylor and Francis Group. Reprinted by permission.

TABLE 3.10. Spearman Correlations between Ratings of ADHD Symptom Dimensions and Impairment Dimensions

Impairment dimensions	ADHD symptoms		
	Inattention	Hyperactive–Impulsive	Total
Parents			
Family Relations	.47	.41	.49
Peer Relations	.42	.44	.47
Homework	.63*	.37*	.59
Academics	.61*	.35*	.56
Behavior	.51	.52	.56
Self-Esteem	.44*	.34*	.44
Teachers			
Teacher Relations	.59	.60	.63
Peer Relations	.61	.64	.65
Homework	.76*	.54*	.73
Academics	.82*	.57*	.78
Behavior	.71*	.77*	.77
Self-Esteem	.60*	.50*	.60

Note. All correlations significant at $p < .001$. *Difference in correlations between the impairment dimensions and the symptom dimensions (Inattention vs. Hyperactivity–Impulsivity) significant ($p < .001$). From Power et al. (2015). Copyright 2015 by Taylor and Francis Group. Reprinted by permission.

IA symptoms and impairments than between HI symptoms and impairments on the Academic, Homework, and Self-Esteem impairment factors (see Table 3.10). Regardless of symptom dimension, correlations between symptom and impairment dimensions were stronger for teachers than for parents ($p < .001$ for all comparisons; median of .61 for teachers vs. .44 for parents).

Each area of impairment was found to have moderate to high correlations with IA symptom ratings according to both parent and teacher report. Not surprisingly, Academic and Homework impairments had the strongest correlations with IA symptoms for both respondents. Correlations between Inattention and Academic/Homework impairment were higher than found for HI and Academic/Homework impairment. This is consistent with many research studies showing a strong link between Inattention and academic performance (e.g., Langberg et al., 2011). Moderate to high correlations between impairment and HI symptoms were also found for teacher ratings, with strongest correlations obtained for Behavior Problems, Peer Relations, and Teacher Relations. Thus, as has been found previously, HI symptoms have a strong relationship with behavior control and social interactions (Nigg, 2001). Overall, correlations between ADHD symptoms and impairment were stronger for teacher than for parent ratings, especially with respect to HI symptoms. It is possible that ADHD symptoms are more impairing in the structured school environment, where self-regulation demands are higher and students are expected to complete academic tasks and follow classroom rules for extended periods. Alternatively, teachers may be in a better position to judge level of impairment because teachers typically have greater experience than parents in making normative comparisons.

Gender, Age, and Racial/Ethnic Group Differences

Our work with the prior version of this scale (i.e., ADHD Rating Scale–IV) indicated that IA, HI, and total scores may vary as a function of child demographic characteristics, including gender, age, and race/ethnicity (DuPaul, Anastopoulos, et al., 1998; DuPaul et al., 1997). Furthermore, it is possible that scores could vary as a function of teacher race/ethnicity. Thus we conducted a series of analyses to examine the degree to which ADHD symptom and impairment ratings differed as a function of child and teacher characteristics. For impairment ratings, we also examined the degree to which IA and HI symptom scores predicted impairment scores above and beyond child demographic factors. Stated differently, we were interested in the degree to which child symptoms contributed to impairment beyond potential gender, age, and race/ethnicity effects.

Symptom Ratings on the ADHD Rating Scale–5

Sum scores for parent and teacher ratings on the ADHD Rating Scale–5 were computed with unit weights for the 18 symptom items (Wainer, 1976). A 2 (Child Gender) × 4 (Child Age groups: 5–7, 8–10, 11–13, and 14–17) × 4 (Child Race/Ethnicity: non-Hispanic white, non-Hispanic African American, Asian, Hispanic) factor analysis of covariance (ANCOVA) was used to assess differences in sum scores for parent ratings on each factor across child demographic groups while controlling for household income. A 2 × 4 × 4 analysis of variance (ANOVA) was used to assess differences for teacher ratings; measures of household income were not available as a covariate for teacher ratings. In addition, a 3 (Student Race/Ethnicity: non-Hispanic white, non-Hispanic African American, Hispanic) × 3 (Teacher Race/Ethnicity: non-Hispanic white, non-Hispanic African American, Hispanic) ANCOVA was used to estimate the interaction between the child and teacher race/ethnicity while controlling for student gender and age. Asian students were excluded from the latter ANCOVA due to small cell size when crossed with teacher race/ethnicity. For these sets of analyses, the alpha level was set at .01 to account for the number of tests conducted. Cohen's *d* was computed for specific comparisons between two groups (i.e., gender), and partial eta squared (η_p^2) for comparisons between three or more groups (i.e., race/ethnicity and age). Partial eta-squared can be interpreted as the proportion of variance explained by the factor after controlling for the other factors in a factor ANCOVA or ANOVA. Cohen's *d* estimates for the parent ratings were computed based on covariate-adjusted means (i.e., controlling for family income) and the mean square error of the ANCOVA.

Parent Symptom Ratings

There were statistically significant two-way (gender × age) interaction effects for the total score (F [3, 1991] = 4.43, $p < .01$, $\eta_p^2 = .007$) and the IA score (F [3, 1992] = 3.87, $p < .01$, $\eta_p^2 = .006$). For the gender × age interactions, post hoc tests indicated that males received higher scores compared to females for the youngest three age groups; however, females in the 14–17 age group received slightly higher scores than males for both scores. The main effects of gender were significant for the total score (F [1, 1991] = 6.90, $p < .01$, $d = 0.17$ [95% CI = 0.08, 0.25]), where males received higher scores than females. The main effect for gender on HI ($p = 0.023$, $d = 0.18$) was not statistically significant at the adjusted level.

There were significant main effects of age on the total score (F [3, 1991] = 3.95, $p < .01$, $\eta_p^2 = .006$) and the HI score (F [3, 1991] = 14.36, $p < .001$, $\eta_p^2 = .021$). Post hoc tests revealed that the youngest children (ages 5–7) received higher scores than children in the oldest age group (ages 14–17) on the total score, and that children in the oldest group received significantly lower scores than children in the two youngest groups (ages 5–10) on HI. Lastly, the main effects of race/ethnicity were significant for the total score (F [3, 1991] = 5.11, $p < .01$, $\eta_p^2 = .008$), IA score (F [3, 1992] = 4.20, $p < .01$, $\eta_p^2 = .006$), and the HI score (F [3, 1991] = 5.12, $p < .001$, $\eta_p^2 = .008$) (see Figures 3.1 and 3.2 for mean scores across racial/ethnic groups for boys and girls, respectively). For the total score, non-Hispanic African American ($d = 0.22$ [0.07, 0.37]) and non-Hispanic white children ($d = 0.22$ [0.11, 0.33]) had higher scores than Hispanic children; for the IA score, non-Hispanic white children received higher scores than Hispanic children ($d = 0.21$ [0.10, 0.31]); and for the HI score, non-Hispanic African American ($d = 0.25$ [0.11, 0.40]) and white children ($d = 0.20$ [0.09, 0.31]) received higher scores than Hispanic children.

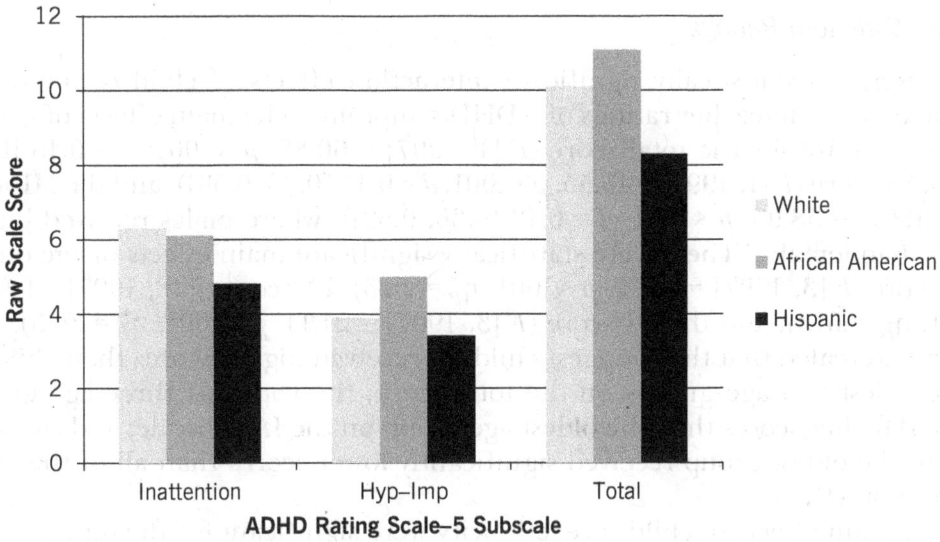

FIGURE 3.1. Mean ADHD Rating Scale–5 Inattention, Hyperactivity–Impulsivity, and Total scores as a function of race/ethnicity for boys, based on parent report.

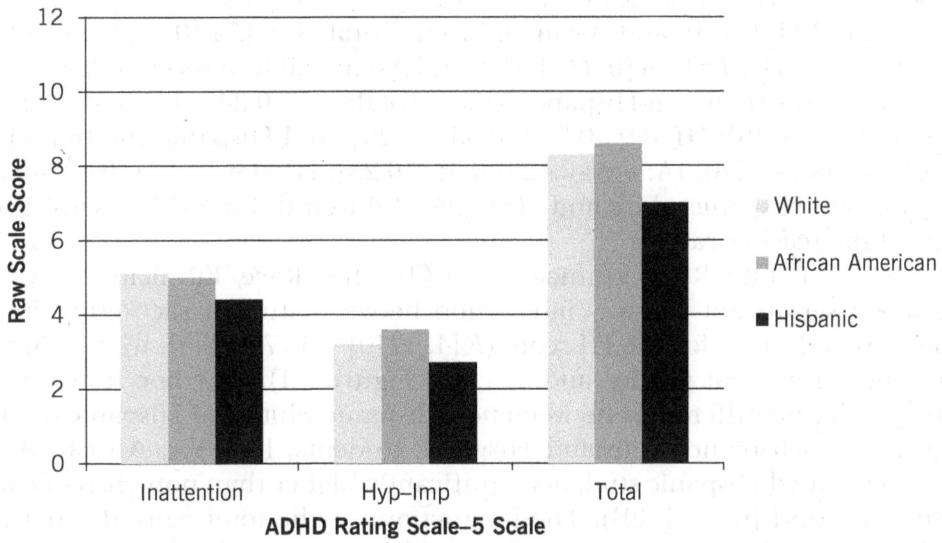

FIGURE 3.2. Mean ADHD Rating Scale–5 Inattention, Hyperactivity–Impulsivity, and Total scores as a function of race/ethnicity for girls, based on parent report.

Teacher Symptom Ratings

There were no statistically significant interaction effects of child demographic characteristics on teacher ratings of ADHD symptoms. The main effects of gender were significant for the total score (F [1, 1997] = 60.83, $p < .001$, d = 0.48 [0.39, 0.56]), IA score (F [1, 1997] = 45.55, $p < .001$, d = 0.44 [0.36, 0.53]), and the HI score (F [1, 1997] = 58.99, $p < .001$, d = 0.43 [0.35, 0.52]), where males received higher scores than females. There were statistically significant main effects of age on the total score (F [3, 1997] = 16.75, $p < .001$, $\eta^2_p = .025$), IA score (F [3, 1997] = 9.00, $p < .001$, $\eta^2_p = .013$), and the HI score (F [3, 1997] = 24.14, $p < .001$, $\eta^2_p = .035$). Post hoc tests revealed that the youngest children received higher scores than children in the oldest two age groups on the total score; the youngest three age groups received higher scores than the oldest age group on the IA subscale; and that children in the oldest group received significantly lower scores than all of the other children on HI.

The main effects of child race/ethnicity were significant for the total score (F [3, 1997] = 24.17, $p < .001$, $\eta^2_p = .035$), IA score (F [3, 1997] = 19.03, $p < .001$, $\eta^2_p = .028$), and the HI score (F [3, 1997] = 22.69, $p < .001$, $\eta^2_p = .033$) (see Figures 3.3 and 3.4 for mean scores across racial/ethnic groups for boys and girls, respectively). For all three scores, non-Hispanic African American children received higher scores than non-Hispanic white (Total: d = 0.40 [0.27, 0.53]; IA: d = 0.37 [0.24, 0.50]; HI: d = 0.38 [0.25, 0.51]), Hispanic (Total: d = 0.28 [0.13, 0.42]; IA: d = 0.22 [0.08, 0.37]; HI: d = 0.29 [0.14, 0.44]), and Asian children (Total: d = 0.74 [0.53, 0.95]; IA: d = 0.64 [0.43, 0.84]; HI: d = 0.73 [0.52, 0.94]); and Asian children received lower symptom rating scores than non-Hispanic white (Total: d = –0.34 [–0.52, –0.17]; IA: d = –0.28 [–0.45, –0.10]; HI: d = –0.37 [–0.55, –0.20]) and Hispanic children (Total: d = –0.47 [–0.66, –0.28]; IA: d = –0.42 [–0.61, –0.23]; HI: d = –0.45 [–0.63, –0.26]). Scores for non-Hispanic white and Hispanic children did not differ significantly for any of the teacher ratings.

For the 3 (Child Race/Ethnicity) × 3 (Teacher Race/Ethnicity) ANCOVA, there was a significant two-way interaction between student race/ethnicity and teacher race/ethnicity for the HI score (F [4, 1740] = 3.77, $p < .01$, $\eta^2_p = .005$) while controlling for student gender and age (see Figure 3.1). Post hoc tests revealed that there were no differences between non-Hispanic white and Hispanic teachers' ratings of non-Hispanic white and Hispanic students; however, African American teachers rated Hispanic students significantly higher than non-Hispanic white students (d = 0.84 [0.38, 1.30]). The interaction for the total score did not meet the adjusted significance level (F [4, 1740] = 2.83, $p = .049$, $\eta^2_p = .005$), but teachers exhibited the same pattern of ratings as for the HI score. There was a significant main effect of teacher race/ethnicity for the HI score (F [2, 1740] = 10.64, $p < .01$, $\eta^2_p = .012$) with non-Hispanic white teachers providing significantly lower scores compared to both non-Hispanic African American (d = –0.24 [–0.45, –0.03]) and Hispanic teachers (d = –0.33 [–0.49, –0.16]). Scores provided by non-Hispanic African American and Hispanic teachers did not differ significantly. No significant interactions or main effects were found for IA scores.

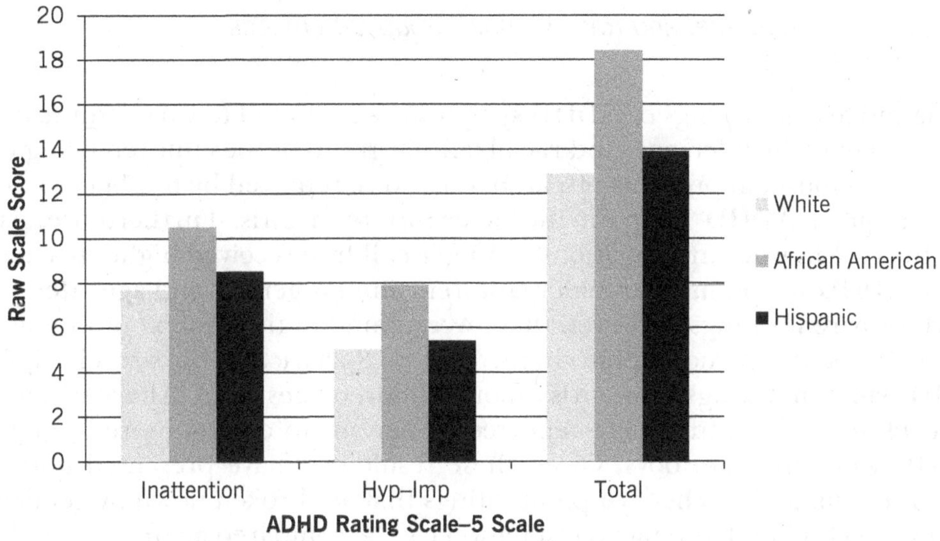

FIGURE 3.3. Mean ADHD Rating Scale–5 Inattention, Hyperactivity–Impulsivity, and Total scores as a function of race/ethnicity for boys, based on teacher report.

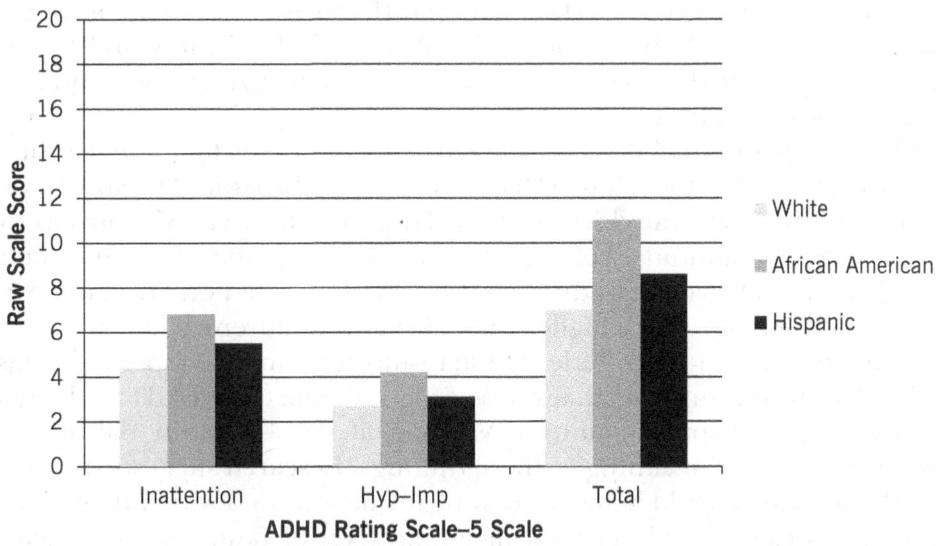

FIGURE 3.4. Mean ADHD Rating Scale–5 Inattention, Hyperactivity–Impulsivity, and Total scores as a function of race/ethnicity for girls, based on teacher report.

Summary of Gender, Age, and Racial/Ethnic Group Differences on Symptom Ratings

Parent and teacher ratings of ADHD symptoms were found to vary significantly as a function of the gender, age, and racial/ethnic group of the children being rated. As has been found in previous research, boys were reported by teachers to exhibit more frequent ADHD symptomatic behaviors than girls. Furthermore, as has been the case in prior investigations, younger children received higher teacher ratings of ADHD symptoms than older children. Similar gender and age effects were found for parent ratings; however, these were found in the context of interactions between these two demographic characteristics. Specifically, boys received higher ADHD symptom ratings than girls among children ages 5–13. Alternatively, girls in the 14- to 17-year range were reported by parents to exhibit more frequent IA and HI symptoms than boys. Given these results, we have presented normative data for parent and teacher symptom ratings that are broken down by gender and age. Thus a child undergoing an evaluation can be compared against norms based on that child's gender and age.

The pattern of findings related to child race/ethnic group differences varied by informant. Teachers rated non-Hispanic African American children higher than non-Hispanic white, Asian, and Hispanic children for inattention and hyperactivity–impulsivity. Effects associated with racial/ethnic group were small to medium in magnitude. These group differences are consistent with those derived for the ADHD Rating Scale–IV (DuPaul et al., 1997). Research is needed to understand factors that account for higher teacher ratings for non-Hispanic African American children.

Findings regarding child race/ethnicity were different for parent ratings of ADHD symptoms. For the total ADHD score, non-Hispanic African American and white children were rated higher than Hispanic children. This group difference was small in magnitude. For the IA scale, non-Hispanic white children were rated higher than Hispanic children, and on the HI scale non-Hispanic African American children were rated higher than Hispanic children. These group differences were also small in magnitude. These results for parent symptom ratings are consistent with recent findings that rates of parent-reported ADHD are higher for non-Hispanic than Hispanic children (Visser et al., 2014). Additional research is needed to explicate the meaning of these findings. Research suggests that perceptions of the severity of child behavior may be influenced by a wide range of family, cultural, and socioeconomic factors, including level of family stress, single parent status, number of children in the home, level of acculturation, and culturally influenced thresholds for differentiating normal from abnormal behavior (Cauce et al., 2002; Eiraldi, Mazzuca, Clarke, & Power, 2006).

We were also able to examine the degree to which teacher race/ethnicity affected ADHD symptom ratings both alone and in combination with child race/ethnicity. Teacher ratings of inattention symptoms were very consistent; there were no main effects of teacher race/ethnicity and no student–teacher interaction effects of race/ethnicity on IA scores. This finding is consistent with research demonstrating the similarity of teacher ratings and direct observations of classroom behavior for children of diverse racial groups (Epstein et al., 2005). With regard to HI symptom ratings, most of the interaction effects examined were not statistically significant, suggesting that teachers of varying racial/ethnic backgrounds generally rated students of diverse backgrounds similarly. An exception to this rule is that African American teachers rated Hispanic students significantly higher than non-Hispanic white students. This group difference was associated with a large effect size. Further, the findings uncovered a tendency for non-Hispanic white teachers to rate HI symptoms lower than Hispanic and non-Hispanic African American teachers regardless of child racial/ethnic group, although effects sizes were small. The tendency for Hispanic teachers to report higher ratings of HI symptoms than white teachers is consistent with the findings of deRamirez and Shapiro (2005), although the latter investigators found this difference only when teachers rated Hispanic students. Replication of these findings is needed, especially given that some cell sizes in the analyses of interaction effects were relatively small. Furthermore, we are unable to provide separate norms for each child racial/ethnic group owing to insufficient cell size within gender and age groups. Thus, although our normative data are representative of the U.S. population with respect to race/ethnicity, clinicians should be cautious in using these data when evaluating teacher ratings of African American children so as to avoid overidentification of them as having ADHD.

Impairment Ratings on the ADHD Rating Scale–5

Impairment ratings were categorical (i.e., derived from 4-point scale) and nonnormally distributed, so their use as dependent variables violate assumptions of parametric linear models (DeMaris, 2013). Thus analyses of impairment ratings were conducted with nonparametric methods, specifically relationships between child demographic characteristics, symptom ratings, and impairment ratings were explored through logistic regression.

In testing logistic regression models, discrimination can be quantified by the area under the receiver operating characteristic curve (AUC), where values smaller than 0.70 represent poor discrimination, values of 0.70–0.79 represent adequate discrimination, values of 0.80–0.89 represent excellent discrimination, and values above 0.89 represent outstanding discrimination (DeMaris, 2013). Predictive effect size can be quantified by odds ratios and McFadden's pseudo R^2. Odds ratios estimate the effect of individual predictors on the criterion whereas the pseudo R^2 is useful in comparing models as additional predictors are added. Higher pseudo R^2 values indicate better prediction accuracy, with R^2 values less than 0.1 considered weak (Garson, 2014) and values of 0.2 to 0.4 identified as satisfactory (Petrucci, 2009).

The multivariate relationships of child gender, age, ethnicity/race, ADHD symptom ratings, and impairment ratings were examined with Stata 13 for Mac. Independent variables in the regression analyses included the demographic characteristics of child gender (males as reference level), age (continuous), race/ethnicity (white non-Hispanics as reference level), and mean item scores on the IA and HI symptom factors.

Given the findings from the confirmatory factor analyses (see Chapter 2) for the impairment items indicating that the optimal model had six factors, each consisting of the two items pertaining to impairment due to IA and HI corresponding with the six areas of impairment assessed, these factors served as dependent variables in the logistic models. To reduce sparseness, the "or" rule, which is commonly used in assessment to resolve discrepancies in ratings (e.g., Shemmassian & Lee, 2012), was applied to determine an individual's score on each impairment factor. The score for a child was 1 if either the IA *or* HI impairment item indicated moderate to severe impairment. The score was 0 if the IA *and* HI impairment items were both rated as none to minor impairment.

As displayed in Table 3.11, parent and teacher impairment ratings were affected by demographic factors (child gender, age, and race/ethnicity); however, the effect sizes were weak (pseudo R^2 = .01 to .07) and group discrimination (AUC = .56 to .69) was poor. The incremental effect of ADHD symptom scores (over and above the effect of demographic variables) was analyzed with a second logistic regression model. All logistic regression models were significantly improved by the addition of ADHD ratings as predictors. The resulting effect sizes were satisfactory (pseudo R^2 = .23 to .55) and group discrimination (AUC = .88 to .95) was excellent to outstanding.

The unique contribution of each demographic factor to binary ratings of impairment is presented in Table 3.12. The findings indicated a significant effect

TABLE 3.11. Global Comparison of Models with Demographic Factors Only (Child Gender, Age, and Ethnicity/Race) to Models with Demographic Factors and ADHD Symptom Scores (Inattention and Hyperactivity–Impulsivity) across Binary Impairment Ratings

	Demographic factors				+ ADHD symptoms				Difference	
Criterion	X^2	*df*	R^2	AUC	X^2	*df*	R^2	AUC	ΔX^2	*df*
Parents										
Family Relations	7.8	5	.01	.56	362*	7	.30	.89	354.6*	2
Peer Relations	7.8	5	.01	.57	301*	7	.31	.90	293.4*	2
Homework	60.9*	5	.04	.66	611*	7	.43	.93	550.1*	2
Academic	52.6*	5	.04	.65	591*	7	.43	.93	538.6*	2
Behavior	27.3*	5	.03	.63	426*	7	.43	.94	399.6*	2
Self-Esteem	10.3	5	.01	.58	290*	7	.28	.88	280.2*	2
Teachers										
Teacher Relations	50.8*	5	.03	.63	656.1*	7	.40	.92	605.3*	2
Peer Relations	79.3*	5	.05	.66	738.7*	7	.43	.92	659.4*	2
Homework	71.0*	5	.03	.61	1068*	7	.42	.91	997.2*	2
Academic	76.8*	5	.03	.62	1375*	7	.52	.94	1298.9*	2
Behavior	159.7*	5	.07	.69	1228*	7	.55	.95	1069.2*	2
Self-Esteem	45.1*	5	.02	.62	537*	7	.30	.88	492.2*	2

Note. R^2 is McFadden's pseudo R^2; AUC is the area under the receiver operating characteristic (ROC); and ΔX^2 is the difference in the log likelihood test of the demographic model versus the demographic + ADHD symptoms model. From Power et al. (2015). Copyright 2015 by Taylor and Francis Group. Reprinted by permission.

$^*p < .001$.

TABLE 3.12. Effects of Child Gender, Age, and Race/Ethnicity on Binary Impairment Ratings

	Gender		Age		Ethnicity/race					
					Black		Hispanic		Other	
Criterion	z	OR	z	OR	z	OR	z	OR	z	OR
Parents										
Family Relations	1.45	1.31 [0.91–1.88]	1.67	1.04 [0.99–1.09]	0.51	1.18 [0.62–2.25]	–1.08	0.76 [0.46–1.25]	–0.44	0.88 [0.49–1.56]
Peer Relations	–1.00	0.80 [0.53–1.23]	1.31	1.04 [0.98–1.10]	1.29	1.58 [0.79–3.14]	–1.27	0.72 [0.43–1.20]	–0.71	0.77 [0.37–1.60]
Homework	–3.19*	0.57 [0.41–.081]	4.26*	1.10 [1.05–1.15]	0.48	1.15 [0.64–2.07]	–1.16	0.77 [0.50–1.20]	–1.02	0.75 [0.43–1.31]
Academic	–2.14	0.68 [0.48–0.97]	3.61*	1.09 [1.04–1.14]	2.18	1.82 [1.06–3.13]	–0.76	0.84 [0.54–1.31]	–0.73	0.81 [0.46–1.43]
Behavior	–2.66*	0.55 [0.35–0.85]	–2.41	0.94 [0.89–0.99]	2.44	2.14 [1.16–3.95]	0.25	1.07 [0.62–1.84]	–0.11	0.96 [0.48–1.90]
Self-Esteem	–0.42	0.92 [0.62–1.36]	2.01	1.05 [1.00–1.10]	–0.07	0.97 [0.45–2.10]	–0.63	0.86 [0.54–1.38]	–0.19	0.94 [0.50–1.77]
Teacher										
Teacher Relations	–3.83*	0.52 [0.37–0.73]	–1.20	0.97 [0.93–1.02]	2.66	1.81 [1.17–2.80]	1.06	1.24 [0.83–1.86]	–2.26	0.42 [0.19–0.89]
Peer Relations	–3.85*	0.51 [0.36–0.72]	–5.06*	0.89 [0.85–0.93]	3.03	1.95 [1.26–2.99]	–0.19	0.96 [0.63–1.46]	–2.12	0.38 [0.16–0.93]
Homework	–5.51*	0.50 [0.39–0.64]	–0.04	1.00 [0.97–1.03]	2.91	1.72 [1.19–2.49]	2.49	1.44 [1.08–1.92]	–1.24	0.72 [0.43–1.21]
Academic	–4.93*	0.55 [0.44–0.70]	–2.01	0.97 [0.94–1.00]	4.44*	2.18 [1.54–3.07]	2.30	1.39 [1.05–1.85]	–0.63	0.86 [0.53–1.38]
Behavior	–7.04*	0.37 [0.28–0.48]	–6.03*	0.89 [0.85–0.92]	4.09*	2.21 [1.51–3.24]	–0.36	0.94 [0.67–1.32]	–2.77	0.39 [0.20–0.76]
Self-Esteem	–3.31*	0.59 [0.43–0.81]	–2.89	0.94 [0.90–0.98]	1.71	1.44 [0.95–2.18]	1.10	1.23 [0.85–1.78]	–2.41	0.41 [0.20–0.85]

Note. Male is the reference category for Gender; Ethnicity/race = white non-Hispanic (the reference category), black non-Hispanic, Hispanic, and other; OR is the odds ratio; IN is Inattention; HI is Hyperactivity–Impulsivity; the 95% confidence interval of OR is in brackets. From Power et al. (2015). Copyright 2015 by Taylor and Francis Group. Reprinted by permission.

$^*p < .001$.

of gender for parent ratings of Homework and Behavior Problems and teacher ratings for all areas of impairment. The odds ratios ranged from 0.37 to 0.57, suggesting effect sizes in the small to medium range. The effect of age was less striking (small effect sizes); the findings indicated that higher age was associated with significantly *higher* impairment for parent ratings of Homework and Academic Problems and significantly *lower* impairment for teacher ratings of Peer Relationships and Behavior Problems. Racial/ethnic group membership generally did not have an effect on ratings of impairment, with the exception that black children were rated significantly higher than non-Hispanic white children for Academic and Behavior Problems, with small to moderate effect sizes.

Given that the global models exhibited predictive and discriminative utility, the multivariate effects of each symptom dimension were subsequently analyzed (see Table 3.13). In contrast to child demographic factors, which generally had weak effects on ratings of impairment, parent and teacher ratings of IA and HI symptoms were powerful predictors of impairment.

Parent ratings of IA symptoms were significantly related to all six impairment dimensions and ratings of HI symptoms were significantly related to Family Relationships, Peer Relationships, and Behavior Problems impairment dimensions. Inattention had uniquely negative effects on Homework and Academic impairment dimensions. For example, for every unit increase in ratings of IA symptoms, the odds of a child being rated as academically impaired were 16.60 times greater, holding all other variables constant.

TABLE 3.13. Effects of Inattention and Hyperactivity–Impulsivity Symptom Scores on Binary Impairment Ratings with Child Demographic Variables Included in the Model

	ADHD symptom score			
	Inattention		Hyperactivity-Impulsivity	
Criterion	*z*	OR	*z*	OR
Parent ratings				
Family Relations	5.86*	3.12 [2.13–4.56]	5.77*	4.17 [2.57–6.77]
Peer Relations	4.26*	2.65 [1.68–4.09]	4.80*	3.66 [2.15–6.21]
Homework	10.80*	14.91 [9.13–24.34]	-1.18	0.75 [0.47–1.21]
Academics	10.95*	16.60 [10.04–27.45]	-1.02	0.78 [0.49–1.26]
Behavior	5.86*	4.00 [2.52–6.36]	6.28*	5.42 [3.20–9.18]
Self-Esteem	7.87*	4.40 [3.04–6.36]	2.07	1.59 [1.02–2.47]
Teacher ratings				
Teacher Relations	9.77*	4.40 [3.27–5.92]	5.51*	2.81 [1.95–4.06]
Peer Relations	7.19*	3.49 [2.48–4.91]	8.60*	5.12 [3.53–7.43]
Homework	13.27*	13.43 [9.15–19.71]	0.30	1.06 [0.73–1.53]
Academics	13.59*	35.92 [21.43–60.22]	-2.21	0.64[0.42–0.95]
Behavior	8.53*	3.52 [2.64–4.70]	11.80*	13.31 [8.66–20.47]
Self-Esteem	11.72*	4.83 [3.71–6.29]	2.03	1.40 [1.01–1.94]

Note. OR is the odds ratio; the 95% confidence interval of the OR is in brackets. From Power et al. (2015).

*$p < .001$.

Teacher ratings of Inattention symptoms significantly affected all six impairment dimensions, whereas ratings of HI symptoms significantly affected only Teacher Relationships, Peer Relationships, and Behavior Problems impairment dimensions. Similar to parent reports, ratings of IA symptoms had uniquely negative effects on Homework and Academic impairment dimensions. As an example, for every unit increase in ratings of IA symptoms, the odds of a child being rated as academically impaired were 35.92 times greater, holding all other variables constant.

Given that symptom counts often are used clinically in the assessment of ADHD, the relationship of impairment ratings and elevations in ADHD symptom counts was also examined with logistic regression. Logistic models were fitted with the six binary impairment indicators serving as dependent variables and elevations in symptom counts serving as the sole predictor. Elevations in symptom counts were determined by classifying children into the (1) Inattention presentation category if they received ratings of often or very often on six or more IA items; (2) Hyperactivity–Impulsivity presentation category if they received ratings of often or very often on six or more HI items; and (3) Combined presentation category if they received ratings of often or very often on six or more items on each symptom dimension.

Results for parent and teacher respondents are presented in Table 3.14. For parents, all impairment dimensions were significantly predicted by elevated ADHD symptom counts (i.e., $\geq$ 6 symptoms endorsed on an ADHD symptom dimension) with satisfactory effect sizes (pseudo R^2 = .17 to .33) and adequate to excellent group discrimination (AUC = .72 to .83). Elevations in symptom counts were associated with significant differences on each impairment dimension. Homework and Academic impairments were most strongly affected by Inattention presentation. In contrast, the Behavior dimension of impairment was most powerfully affected by the Hyperactive–Impulsive and Combined presentations. The odds of being rated as having a behavioral impairment were 88.51 times larger if there were parent-rated elevations for Hyperactive–Impulsive or Combined presentations than if the child did not meet symptom criteria for ADHD, holding other variables constant.

For teachers, all impairment dimensions were significantly predicted by elevations in ADHD symptom count with satisfactory effect sizes (pseudo R^2 = .23 to .37) and adequate to excellent group discrimination (AUC = .77 to .84). Similar to findings for parent ratings, Homework and Academic impairments were most powerfully affected by elevations on Inattention. In contrast, all impairment dimensions were strongly affected by the presence of elevations on both dimensions of ADHD (i.e., Combined presentation). Holding all other variables constant, children meeting symptom criteria for Combined presentation had a much higher risk of impairment than those not meeting criteria for ADHD: 210.59 times larger for Behavior Problems, 53.25 times larger for Peer Relationships, 48.71 times larger for Teacher Relationships, and 42.00 times larger for Academics. For both parent and teacher ratings, children with symptom ratings consistent with ADHD diagnostic presentations were statistically and clinically different on all impairment dimensions when compared to children whose symptom ratings were not consistent with ADHD diagnoses.

TABLE 3.14. Logistic Regressions Predicting Binary Impairment Dimension Scores from Clinically Relevant Elevations in ADHD Symptom Counts (Inattention, Hyperactivity–Impulsivity, and Combined) for Parents and Teachers

					ADHD dimension[a]					
					IN		HI		Combined	
Criterion	X^2	*df*	R^2	AUC	*z*	OR	*z*	OR	*z*	OR
Parents										
Family Relations	216.5*	3	.18	.72	7.60*	7.64	4.81*	8.48	11.5*	31.62
Peer Relations	199.8*	3	.21	.75	8.35*	8.48	5.89*	11.20	13.2*	34.09
Homework	355.5*	3	.25	.76	15.39*	23.66	2.84*	3.70	13.2*	30.70
Academic	354.6*	3	.26	.77	15.57*	25.41	3.06*	4.11	13.2*	30.42
Behavior	322.4*	3	.33	.83	9.72*	13.22	8.98*	30.68	15.4*	88.51
Self-Esteem	176.6	3	.17	.73	10.36*	10.73	3.61*	5.37	11.4*	19.93
Teachers										
Teacher Relations	505.8*	3	.31	.84	13.65*	13.31	8.31*	14.19	18.9*	48.71
Peer Relations	537.9*	3	.32	.83	12.25*	9.72	10.33*	22.52	19.4*	53.26
Homework	654.2*	3	.26	.77	18.05*	19.42	5.59*	4.91	15.8*	25.91
Academic	827.4*	3	.31	.78	17.40*	43.91	3.53*	2.82	14.8*	42.00
Behavior	835.2*	3	.37	.83	15.66*	11.28	10.70*	34.71	15.1*	210.59
Self-Esteem	417.1*	3	.23	.78	14.96*	11.39	6.28*	7.06	16.5*	20.32

Note. R^2 is McFadden's pseudo R^2; AUC is the area under the receiver operating characteristic (ROC); OR is the odds ratio; IN, Inattention; HI, Hyperactivity–Impulsivity. From Power et al. (2015). Copyright 2015 by Taylor and Francis Group. Reprinted by permission.

[a]Reference level is non-ADHD.

$^*p < .001$.

Summary of Impact of Gender, Age, Race/Ethnicity, and Symptom Ratings on Impairment Ratings

Although associations between child characteristics and impairment ratings were relatively weak, they were generally consistent with the results of prior investigations, especially for gender and race/ethnicity. Child gender significantly predicted all areas of impairment rated by teachers and Homework and Behavior Problems rated by parents. These findings confirm the results of other studies showing relatively large differences in ADHD symptom frequency between boys and girls (e.g., Polanczyk, de Lima, Horta, Biederman, & Rohde, 2007) as well as recent findings that high school teachers rate boys as having more impairment than girls (Evans et al., 2013). In contrast, race/ethnicity generally was not a significant predictor of any area of impairment other than teacher ratings of Academics and Behavior Problems for black versus non-Hispanic white children. Follow-up sensitivity analyses further revealed that socioeconomic status, assessed by parental level of education, was not related to level of impairment as rated by parents. The findings for teacher ratings are consistent with those of prior studies showing differences in ADHD symptom ratings across racial/ethnic groups (e.g., Reid et al., 1998), higher teacher impairment ratings for African American versus white high school students (Evans et al., 2013), and previous studies highlighting racial/ethnic differences in academic achievement (e.g., Fryer & Levitt, 2004).

Child age was a significant predictor of impairment ratings in two areas (Homework, Academics) for parents and two different areas (Peer Relations, Behavior Problems) for teachers. Consistent with typical findings of higher Inattention, Hyperactivity–Impulsivity, and total ADHD symptom ratings for younger children (e.g., DuPaul et al., 1997; Reynolds & Kamphaus, 2004), older age in this study was associated with lower teacher ratings of symptom-related impairment. In contrast to previous findings for symptom ratings, older age was associated with higher parent ratings of symptom-related impairment. These findings suggest that although ADHD-related behaviors may be more frequent among younger children, the impact of symptomatic behaviors is of greater concern to parents for older children and adolescents, especially in the areas of Homework and Academic functioning. In conclusion, child demographic factors demonstrated associations with ratings of impairment but the relationships generally were weak. These associations were reduced when symptom ratings were included in multivariate models.

One major conclusion from our analyses of impairment ratings is that these scores are more directly affected by ADHD symptoms than by child demographic characteristics. Specifically, although child gender, age, and race/ethnicity significantly predicted ratings of impairment in Homework, Behavior Problems, and Academics (for both respondents) as well as ratings of impairment in Teacher Relations, Peer Relations, and Self-Esteem (for teachers), their contributions to increasing model fit (i.e., between .02 and .07) were much lower than found for symptom ratings (i.e., between .28 and .55). Thus ADHD symptom frequency affects parent and teacher ratings of academic, social, and behavioral impairment above and beyond the influence of child characteristics known to affect performance in these areas. Furthermore, symptom ratings representing the combination of both ADHD dimensions were associated with a marked increment in impairment compared to IA or HI symptom ratings alone, particularly for impairment in Family/Teacher Relations, Peer Relations, and Behavior Problems.

Epidemiology of ADHD Presentations

Overall Prevalence

In view of the many circumstances that can affect the outcome of epidemiological research (e.g., sample, diagnostic criteria, assessment procedures, and source of symptom estimates), it is no wonder that there has been a tremendous amount of variability in the ADHD prevalence estimates that have been reported in the literature. For example, among the many studies utilizing DSM-III and DSM-III-R conceptualizations of ADHD, prevalence rates have ranged from as low as 2–3% up to 25–30% of the general child population. Relatively similar findings have been found in studies examining ADHD prevalence based on DSM-IV criteria (for meta-analytic review, see Willcutt, 2012). ADHD prevalence rates are consistently higher when based on teacher symptom ratings relative to parent symptom ratings (teacher-reported prevalence M = 13.3%; 95% CI = 11.6 to 15.2%; parent-reported prevalence M = 8.8%; 95% CI = 7.7 to 9.9%). Importantly, prevalence rates drop markedly when impairment is considered along with symptom report. For example, Willcutt's (2012) meta-analytic review found a 47% reduction in teacher-reported prevalence relative to report based on symptoms alone. Specifically, when teacher-reported symptoms and impairment were considered together, mean total prevalence of ADHD was 7.1% (95% CI: 6.6 to 7.5%), with 2.3% (95% CI = 1.7 to 3.2%) identified with ADHD Combined, 1.1% (95% CI = 0.5 to 2.3%) with ADHD Hyperactive–Impulsive, and 3.4% (95% CI = 3.1 to 3.7%) with ADHD Inattentive. Whether this same pattern holds true for the DSM-5 version of ADHD is unclear, owing to the fact that relatively little research has thus far addressed this matter.

Using the normative samples described earlier in this chapter, we sought to estimate prevalence rates of ADHD using DSM-5 criteria based on symptom count alone, impairment count alone, and the combination of symptom and impairment counts. In so doing, we recognize that we are providing an upper limit on these prevalence estimates, given that we have used some (i.e., symptom frequency, impairment) but not all (i.e., exclusionary conditions) of the DSM-5 criteria for establishing a diagnosis ADHD. For any given child, a symptom was considered present if the item score was a 2 or 3 (i.e., reported to occur often or very often, respectively). Conversely, item scores of 0 or 1 indicated symptom absence. Using the symptomatic cutoffs recommended in DSM-5 (i.e., six of nine symptoms of inattention, and/or six of nine symptoms of hyperactivity–impulsivity), the number of children meeting criteria for each of the three presentations of ADHD was determined. Similarly for impairment ratings, impairment for any item was considered present based on ratings of 2 or 3 (i.e., reported to be a moderate or severe problem) and was considered absent based on ratings of 0 or 1 (i.e., reported to be no or minor problem). Given the normative data analysis conducted for impairment ratings (Power et al., 2015), for prevalence rates based on parent ratings, evidence of inattention-related and/or hyperactivity–impulsivity-related impairment was indicated when at least one of the six impairment items for inattention or hyperactivity–impulsivity was counted as present. For prevalence rates based on teacher ratings, evidence of impairment was indicated when at least three of six impairment items for inattention or hyperactivity–impulsivity were counted as present.

Based on ADHD symptom report alone, we found an overall ADHD prevalence rate of 8.3% based on parent ratings on the Home Version (see Table 3.15) and a prevalence rate of 17.3% based on teacher ratings on the School Version (see Table 3.16). These estimates of overall disorder are very similar to findings for the ADHD Rating Scale–IV (DuPaul, Power, Anastopoulos, & Reid, 1998) as well as prevalence rates obtained in prior investigations for parent report using DSM-IV criteria; however, the teacher report prevalence rate here was somewhat higher than in prior studies (Willcutt, 2012). Furthermore, we found the Inattentive presentation to be most prevalent in our samples. Specifically, teacher ratings on the School Version indicated a prevalence of 9.7% for the Inattentive presentation, 2.3% for the Hyperactive–Impulsive presentation, and 5.3% for the Combined presentation. The same pattern was also evident when parents served as informants,

TABLE 3.15. Diagnostic Status Based on Parent-Reported Symptom Count, Impairment Count, and Combined

	No ADHD	ADHD IA	ADHD HI	ADHD C
Symptom	1,895 (91.7%)	103 (5.0%)	23 (1.1%)	46 (2.2%)
Impairment	1,666 (80.5%)	–	–	403 (19.5%)
Symptom + Impairment	1,933 (93.5 %)	75 (3.6%)	19 (0.9%)	41 (2.0%)

Note. Individual symptom percentages and counts are based on 2,067 children. Impairment percentages and counts are based on 2,069 children. IA, inattentive presentation; HI, hyperactive–impulsive presentation; C, combined presentation.

TABLE 3.16. Diagnostic Status Based on Teacher-Reported Symptom Count, Impairment Count, and Combined

	No ADHD	ADHD IA	ADHD HI	ADHD C
Symptom	1,771 (82.7%)	208 (9.7%)	49 (2.3%)	113 (5.3%)
Impairment	1,723 (80.5%)	–	–	417 (19.5%)
Symptom + Impairment	1,864 (87.1%)	146 (6.8%)	29 (1.4%)	101 (4.7%)

Note. Individual symptom and impairment percentages and counts are based on 2,140 students. IA, inattentive presentation; HI, hyperactive–impulsive presentation; C, combined presentation.

with rates of 5.0%, 1.1%, and 2.2% occurring for the Inattentive, Hyperactive–Impulsive, and Combined presentations, respectively.

When considering ADHD impairment report alone, an overall prevalence rate of 19.5% was found for parent report (see Table 3.15) and 19.5% for teacher report (see Table 3.16). As expected, prevalence rates dropped when diagnostic status was based on the combination of symptom and impairment counts. Overall ADHD prevalence was 6.5% for parent report and 12.9% for teacher report (see Tables 3.15 and 3.16, respectively). The Inattentive presentation was the most prevalent (3.6%) for parent report, followed by Combined (2.0%) and Hyperactive–Impulsive (0.9%) presentations. Similar findings were obtained for teacher report with Inattentive presentation being most prevalent (6.8%) followed by Combined (4.7%) and Hyperactive–Impulsive (1.4%) presentations. Thus ADHD prevalence rates are highest when considering impairment report alone, followed by symptom report alone, and then the combined consideration of symptom and impairment report. These results highlight the critical need to consider both symptoms and impairment when evaluating children for possible ADHD.

Age and Gender Effects on Prevalence

When viewed from the perspective of clinical practice, these results are of limited significance because they do not shed light on individual differences. Of the many individual difference variables that may be considered, age and gender are certainly among those that can have a powerful influence on child psychopathology prevalence estimates. Thus we examined ADHD prevalence rates (based on aforementioned symptom plus impairment criteria) across gender and age categories.

Teacher ratings on the School Version resulted in overall prevalence rates of 17.3% for children 5 to 7 years of age, 16.8% for 8- to 10-year-old children, 12.2% for the 11- to 13-year-olds, and 7.5% for those 14 to 17 years of age. When parents served as informants, the overall prevalence rates were 6.5% for 5- to 7-year-old children, 6.1% for 8- to 10-year-old children, 7.8% for 11- to 13-year-old children, and 6.7% for adolescents between 14 and 17 years of age. These results raise the possibility that the overall prevalence of ADHD, as defined by DSM-5 symptom plus impairment criteria, declines with age for teacher ratings but not for parent ratings.

Implicit throughout the preceding discussion is the notion that ADHD changes in its clinical presentation across development. Although this may seem to be a reasonable conclusion, these findings were derived from cross-sectional investigations. Whether these same developmental trends in ADHD status based on DSM-5 criteria would be evident in longitudinal studies is unknown. Until research of this sort is completed, there are at least cross-sectional data available to raise the possibility that developmental trends exist, particularly for teacher ratings.

Along with these age-related effects, gender can also influence not only the overall rate of ADHD, but also the relative prevalence of each presentation. Specifically, parent ratings on the Home Version indicated a ratio of boys to girls of 1.3:1 for the Inattentive presentation, 2.8:1 for the Hyperactive–Impulsive presentation, and 1.2:1 for the Combined presentation. In contrast, the pattern of findings emerged from the teacher ratings, with ratios of 2:1 for the Inattentive presentation, 1.3:1 for the Hyperactive–Impulsive presentation, and 3.4:1 for the Combined presentation, indicated a stronger likelihood for boys to be identified with Inattentive and Combined presentations.

Racial/Ethnic Group Differences in Prevalence Rates

For ratings of DSM-IV ADHD symptoms on the ADHD Rating Scale–IV, race/ethnicity affected prevalence rates in the context of a community-based sample. Teacher ratings on the School Version identified approximately 6.3% of the white children and adolescents as having one of the three major subtypes of ADHD versus a rate of 12.3% among children and adolescents from racial/ethnic minority backgrounds (i.e., African American and Hispanic). Looking at it from a somewhat different perspective, of the total number of children and adolescents identified with any type of ADHD, 43.4% were from racial/ethnic minority backgrounds, even though children and adolescents from minority backgrounds made up only 34.8% of the total teacher-generated sample. Similar findings emerged from parent ratings on the Home Version; however, these findings were based on symptom ratings alone.

We examined differences across racial/ethnic groups in ADHD prevalence based on DSM-5 symptom report plus impairment as defined previously. Teacher ratings on the School Version identified approximately 12.8% of the white non-Hispanic children and adolescents as having one of the three ADHD presentations versus a rate of 20.3% for African American children and adolescents and a rate of 11.3% for children and adolescents from Hispanic backgrounds. Looking at it from a somewhat different perspective, we can say that of the total number of children and adolescents identified with any type of ADHD, 41.7% were from racial/ethnic minority backgrounds, even though racial/ethnic minority children and adolescents made up only 36.7% of the total teacher-generated sample. Additional research of this type is clearly needed to establish a more definitive connection between race/ethnicity and the prevalence of ADHD. Pending the results of further investigations, clinicians should employ caution in using these scales to diagnose children and adolescents from racial/ethnic minority backgrounds, especially those who are African American.

Summary of Prevalence Rates

Prevalence rates derived from our normative samples are higher than the 3–5% prevalence described in DSM-5. This should not be surprising, given that our rates were derived primarily on the basis of the ADHD symptom plus impairment requirement alone and the report of a single informant. Having been determined in this way, such figures very likely include many children and adolescents for whom ADHD would not be diagnosed, owing to the fact that they would not meet all of the other DSM-5 criteria (e.g., display of symptoms across more than one setting, rule-out of other diagnoses). In light of these circumstances, our estimates are perhaps best viewed as *upper limits* in the true prevalence of ADHD within the general population.

Among clinic samples, the Combined presentation appears to be the most commonly encountered subtype category (Willcutt, 2012), whereas the Inattentive presentation occurs most often in community samples, as presented here. Such a difference suggests that a more severe ADHD presentation is what prompts parents and teachers to refer a child for clinical services. Conversely, this also raises the possibility that many children and adolescents with milder forms of ADHD are not receiving services that could decrease their risk for encountering more serious problems. In addition to these referral considerations, many other factors may affect the prevalence of these presentations. According to teachers, younger children display the Combined presentation most often, whereas older children and adolescents are much more likely to be identified with the Inattentive classification. Similar findings have emerged from parent ratings of older children and adolescents (see Barkley, 2015), but parents are much more likely to identify very young children as having the Hyperactive–Impulsive presentation consistent with the DSM-IV field trials. Of additional interest is that the overall prevalence of DSM-5 defined ADHD—that is, the total for all three presentations—seems to decline with age, at least based on teacher report. Although these findings certainly point to the existence of developmental trends, such a conclusion is limited by the fact that it is based on investigations utilizing cross-sectional, rather than longitudinal, designs.

CHAPTER 4
Reliability and Validity

In this chapter, we review the psychometric properties and technical adequacy of the Home and School versions of the ADHD Rating Scale–5. First, a brief description of the samples and procedures used to conduct these analyses is provided. Then, data regarding the internal consistency, test–retest reliability, interrater agreement, and criterion-related validity of both versions of the scale are presented. Finally, to shed further light on the clinical utility of these scales, data are presented on the discriminant and predictive validities of symptom scores on the previous version of this measure (i.e., the ADHD Rating Scale–IV) in the context of clinic-based and school-based evaluations.

Samples, Procedures, and Results: Internal Consistency

The normative samples and data collection procedures described in Chapter 3 were used to examine internal consistency of symptom scores for parent (pp. 16–20) and teacher (pp. 20–22) ratings. Coefficient alphas were calculated to determine the internal consistency of symptom ratings on the ADHD Rating Scale–5, School Version, and its two subscales. Because impairment ratings were calculated as the higher of IA or HI scores in each of the six domains, internal consistency analyses were not conducted for impairment scores. For child symptom ratings (i.e., 5- to 10-year-olds), the following alpha coefficients were obtained: Total score = .97, Inattention = .96, and Hyperactivity–Impulsivity = .95. For adolescent ratings (i.e., 11- to 17-year-olds), obtained alpha coefficients were: Total score = .96, Inattention = .96, and Hyperactivity–Impulsivity = .94.

In similar fashion, coefficient alphas were calculated to determine the internal consistency of symptom ratings on the ADHD Rating Scale–5, Home Version, and its two subscales. For child ratings, the following alpha coefficients were obtained: Total score = .95, Inattention = .93, and Hyperactivity–Impulsivity = .91. For adolescent ratings, obtained alpha coefficients were: Total score = .94, Inattention = .94, and Hyperactivity–Impulsivity = .89. Thus scores on all versions of the scale demonstrate strong internal consistency.

Sample and Procedures: Test–Retest Reliability, Criterion-Related Validity, and Interrater Agreement

Participants

Students were randomly selected from suburban school districts located in eastern Pennsylvania, eastern Nebraska, and southern New Jersey to examine the test–retest reliability, interrater agreement, and criterion-related validity of ADHD symptom and impairment ratings. Participant samples for teacher ratings, parent ratings, direct observations, and combined parent and teacher ratings are described in detail, below.

Teacher Ratings

Complete data for analyzing the test–retest reliability and criterion-related validity of teacher ratings were available for 64 children (37 boys, 27 girls) ranging in age from 5 to 17 years (M = 10.5; SD = 3.4) who attended kindergarten through 12th grade (M = 5.3; SD = 3.4). Participants were predominantly white (n = 53) but also included children of African American (n = 4), Hispanic (n = 5), Asian American (n = 1), and biracial (n = 5) backgrounds. All but three children were placed in general education classrooms. For the validity analyses of teacher ratings, six of the criterion measures involved direct observation of classroom behavior and academic performance for a subsample of 32 students (13 boys, 19 girls) ranging in age from 6 to 11 years (M = 8.1; SD = 1.5) who attended grades 1–5 (M = 2.7; SD = 1.5).

Parent Ratings

Complete test–retest reliability data for parent ratings were available for 34 children (15 boys, 19 girls) who were primarily white (n = 24), ranged in age from 5 to 17 years (M = 10.1; SD = 3.6), and attended kindergarten through 12th grade (M = 4.7; SD = 3.6). Complete criterion-related validity data for parent ratings were available for 45 children (21 boys, 24 girls) who were primarily white (n = 34), ranged in age from 5 to 17 years (M = 10.1; SD = 3.4) who attended kindergarten through 12th grade (M = 4.7; SD = 3.5).

Interrater Agreement

For analysis of interrater agreement, parent and teacher ratings were available for a sample of 41 students (18 boys, 23 girls). These students were predominantly white (n = 32), ranged in age from 5 to 17 years (M = 10.1; SD = 3.6), and attended kindergarten through 12th grade (M = 4.7; SD = 3.6).

Measures

Parents and teachers were asked to provide information about the child being rated, such as gender, grade, age, race, and ethnicity. Teachers completed either the child or adolescent version of the ADHD Rating Scale–5, School Version, the Conners Teacher Rating Scale (CTRS; Conners, 2008), and the Impairment Rating Scale (IRS; Fabiano et al., 2006). Parents completed either the child or adolescent version of the ADHD Rating Scale–5, Home Version, the Conners Parent Rating Scale (CPRS; Conners, 2008), and the IRS.

The classroom behavior of children who were placed in first through fifth grade was observed by a research assistant using the Behavior Observation of Students in Schools (BOSS; Shapiro, 2011). The occurrence of three behaviors (i.e., off-task motor, off-task passive, off-task verbal) was recorded on a partial interval basis using observation intervals of 15 seconds. Two additional behaviors (i.e., active engaged, passive engaged) were recorded on a momentary time sampling basis at the beginning of each observation interval. Each observation session was approximately 30 minutes in length. For each behavior, the percentage of intervals in which the behavior occurred was calculated by dividing the number of intervals in which the behavior occurred by the total number of observation intervals and multiplying the dividend by 100%.

Criterion-related validity was also examined regarding association of symptom and impairment ratings with performance on classroom assignments. Specifically, samples of classwork completed during the week covered by ADHD Rating Scale–5 ratings were examined for percentage correct responses. In cases where work samples were not available, teachers provided grades (in the form of percentage correct) on academic assignments that were completed during the week.

Procedures

Parent and teacher ratings were obtained over a 7-month period in November 2014 to June 2015 (to ensure teacher familiarity with student behavior). Within each of the districts, two to four children (with an attempt to include equivalent numbers of boys and girls) at each grade level were randomly selected to participate. Only children in general education classrooms participated.

Once written parental permission was obtained, parents and teachers were asked to complete the appropriate version of the ADHD Rating Scale–5 on two occasions approximately 6 weeks apart to assess test–retest reliability. The teacher also completed CTRS and IRS on one of the two occasions, and the parent completed CPRS and IRS on one of the two occasions. For all children in first through fifth grade, a research assistant conducted behavioral observations on three separate occasions (i.e., a total of 90 minutes of observation) during one of the two weeks when parents and teachers were due to complete the ADHD Rating Scale–5. Following each observation, the teacher provided information necessary to calculate a percentage correct score (i.e., how much work was completed correctly relative to the amount assigned). A second observer was present for 30% of the observation sessions so that interobserver agreement could be determined. Interobserver agreement was calculated by dividing the number of agreements by the total number of agreements plus disagreements and multiplying the dividend by 100%. Agreement was consistently above 80% and averaged 85% (occurrence), 96% (non-occurrence), and 98% (total) across the five behavioral categories.

Test–Retest Reliability and Interrater Agreement

Child Version Ratings

Test–retest reliability data were obtained for teacher ratings occurring approximately 6 weeks apart. Pearson product–moment correlation coefficients were as follows: Total score = .93, Inattention = .91, and Hyperactivity–Impulsivity = .90. For impairment ratings, test–retest coefficients (using Spearman rho correlations) were Relationships with School Professionals = .84, Relationships with Students = .88, Homework = .71, Academic Functioning = .70, Behavior Functioning = .85, and Self-Esteem = .62.

Test–retest reliability data were obtained for parent ratings occurring approximately 6 weeks apart. Pearson product–moment correlation coefficients were as follows: Total score = .87, Inattention = .80, and Hyperactivity–Impulsivity = .83. For parent ratings of impairment (using Spearman rho correlations), test-retest coefficients were Family Relationships = .68, Peer Relationships = .63, Homework = .75, Academic Functioning = .90, Behavior Functioning = .66, and Self-Esteem = .62.

Interrater agreement coefficients between parent and teacher symptom ratings were in the moderate range, as follows: Total score = .68, Inattention = .77, and Hyperactivity–Impulsivity = .48. Alternatively, Spearman rho correlations were mixed ranging from low to moderate for agreement on impairment ratings with Relationships with Adults = .11, Peer Relationships = .12, Homework = .60, Academic Functioning = .52, Behavior Functioning = .51, and Self-Esteem = .46.

Adolescent Version Ratings

As was the case for child version ratings, test–retest reliability data were obtained for teacher ratings occurring approximately 6 weeks apart. Pearson product–moment correlation coefficients were as follows: Total score = .91, Inattention = .85, and Hyperactivity–Impulsivity = .77. For impairment ratings, test–retest coefficients (Spearman rho correlations) were Relationships with School Professionals = .92, Relationships with Students = .78, Homework = .69, Academic Functioning = .78, Behavior Functioning = .86, and Self-Esteem = .74.

Test–retest reliability data were obtained for parent ratings occurring approximately 6 weeks apart. Pearson product–moment correlation coefficients were as follows: Total score = .66, Inattention = .70, and Hyperactivity–Impulsivity = .61. For parent ratings of impairment, test–retest coefficients (Spearman rho correlations) were Family Relationships = .81, Peer Relationships = .28, Homework = .44, Academic Functioning = .55, Behavior Functioning = .38, and Self-Esteem = .14.

Interrater agreement coefficients between parent and teacher symptom ratings were mixed, as follows: Total score = .38, Inattention = .46, and Hyperactivity–Impulsivity = .01. Similarly, Spearman rho correlations were mixed ranging from low to moderate for agreement on impairment ratings with Relationships with Adults = .25, Peer Relationships = .25, Homework = .47, Academic Functioning = .50, Behavior Functioning = .77, and Self-Esteem = –.06.

Relationships between Teacher ADHD Symptom Ratings and Criterion Measures

Pearson product-moment correlations between ADHD Rating Scale–5, School Version, symptom rating scores and criterion measures are displayed separately for CTRS T-scores (Table 4.1), IRS raw scores (Table 4.2), and classroom behavioral observations and academic performance (Table 4.3). For correlations with CTRS scores, the absolute values of obtained Pearson correlation coefficients ranged from .46 to .89, with all 45 values achieving statistical significance. If a Bonferroni correction is applied to control Type 1 error rate for multiple correlations (i.e., alpha = .001), all 45 of these correlations can be considered statistically significant. As expected, the strongest correlations were found between ADHD

TABLE 4.1. Validity Coefficients for ADHD Rating Scale–5, School Version, Symptom Ratings with Conners Teacher Rating Scale T-Scores

Measure	Inattention	Hyperactivity–Impulsivity	Total
CTRS DSM-Inattentive	.84	.78	.85
CTRS DSM-Hyp–Imp	.76	.89	.84
CTRS ADHD Index	.87	.84	.89
CTRS Inattention	.85	.75	.84
CTRS Hyperactivity	.77	.89	.85
CTRS LE	.84	.72	.83
CTRS LP	.74	.68	.75
CTRS EF	.85	.66	.80
CTRS AG	.49	.53	.54
CTRS PR	.46	.49	.48
CTRS GI	.85	.82	.87
CTRS AN	.86	.74	.85
CTRS AH	.78	.88	.85
CTRS CD	.49	.46	.49
CTRS OD	.49	.58	.55

Note. CTRS, Conners Teacher Rating Scale; LE, Learning Problems/Executive Functioning; LP, Learning Problems; EF, Executive Functioning; AG, Aggression; PR, Peer Relations; GI, Global Index; AN, ADHD Predominantly Inattentive Type; AH, ADHD Predominantly Hyperactive–Impulsive Type; CD, Conduct Disorder; OD, Oppositional Defiant Disorder.

$p < .001$.

TABLE 4.2. Validity Coefficients for ADHD Rating Scale–5, School Version, Symptom Ratings with Impairment Rating Scale Scores

Measure	Inattention	Hyperactivity–Impulsivity	Total
IRS Peers	.70***	.72***	.73***
IRS Best Friend	.09	.09	.10
IRS Teacher	.67***	.60***	.67***
IRS Academic	.89***	.75***	.87***
IRS Classroom	.66***	.68***	.72***
IRS Self-Esteem	.79***	.74***	.79***
IRS Need for Treatment	.88***	.81***	.89***

Note. IRS, Impairment Rating Scale.
***$p < .001$.

Rating Scale–5, School Version, factor scores and CTRS scores on factors related to ADHD (i.e., DSM-Inattentive, DSM-Hyperactive–Impulsive, ADHD Index, Inattention, and Hyperactivity). In fact, ratings of ADHD symptoms on these two measures shared between 58 and 79% of the variance. Further, as expected, Inattention symptom ratings on the ADHD Rating Scale–5 were more strongly related with CTRS attention-related factors (i.e., DSM-Inattentive, Inattention) than with CTRS hyperactive-impulsive-related factors (i.e., DSM-Hyperactive–Impulsive, Hyperactivity). In similar fashion, Hyperactive–Impulsive symptom ratings on the ADHD Rating Scale–5 were more strongly related with CTRS hyperactive–impulsive-related factors (i.e., DSM-Hyperactive–Impulsive, Hyperactivity) than with inattention-related factors (i.e., DSM-Inattentive, Inattention). Large correlations were found for the total symptom score on the ADHD Rating Scale–5 and all ADHD related factors on the CTRS.

Teacher symptom ratings on the ADHD Rating Scale–5 generally were highly correlated with teacher ratings on the IRS (see Table 4.2). Validity coefficients ranged from .09 to .89 with 18 out of 21 correlations significantly greater than 0 after correction for control of Type I error (alpha = .002). Symptom ratings were

TABLE 4.3. Validity Coefficients for ADHD Rating Scale–5, School Version, Symptom Ratings with Direct Observation and Classroom Measures

Measure	Inattention	Hyperactivity–Impulsivity	Total
BOSS Active Engaged	–.29	–.15	–.25
BOSS Passive Engaged	–.07	–.20	–.12
BOSS Off-Task Motor	.50**	.45*	.50**
BOSS Off-Task Passive	.50**	.38*	.47*
BOSS Off-Task Verbal	.24	.21	.23
Percentage Correct	–.17	–.18	–.18

Note.. BOSS, Behavior Observation of Students in Schools.
*$p < .05$; **$p < .01$.

highly correlated with impairment in relationships with peers and teachers, academic functioning, classroom performance, and self-esteem. Inattention symptom ratings were strongly related to IRS Academic, Self-Esteem, and Need for Treatment scores; while Hyperactive–Impulsive symptom ratings were most strongly related to IRS Need for Treatment, Peers, Academic, and Self-Esteem scores. Coefficients were slightly higher for Inattention ratings than for Hyperactive–Impulsive ratings with IRS Academic, Teacher, Self-Esteem, and Need for Treatment scores.

All three symptom rating scores on the ADHD Rating Scale–5, School Version, were significantly correlated with direct observations of classroom off-task motor behavior and off-task passive behavior (see Table 4.3). As expected, negative relationships were found between teacher symptom ratings and academic performance, assessed by scoring students' work samples, but none of these coefficients were statistically significant. Clearly, validity coefficients were much stronger for relationships with teacher ratings on the CTRS and IRS than with direct observations of classroom behavior and performance. This could be due to shared method and source variance as well as the limited time frame samples for classroom observations relative to the period covered by teacher ratings.

Relationships between Parent ADHD Symptom Ratings and Criterion Measures

Pearson product–moment correlations between ADHD Rating Scale–5, Home Version, symptom rating scores and criterion measures are displayed separately for CPRS T-scores (Table 4.4) and IRS raw scores (Table 4.5). For correlations with CPRS scores, the absolute values of obtained Pearson correlation coefficients

TABLE 4.4. Correlation Coefficients between Parent Symptom Ratings on the ADHD Rating Scale–5, Home Version, and Conners Parent Rating Scale T-Scores

Measure	Inattention	Hyperactivity–Impulsivity	Total
CPRS DSM-Inattentive	.78***	.54***	.70***
CPRS DSM-Hyp–Imp	.65***	.83***	.82***
CPRS ADHD Index	.70***	.76***	.80***
CPRS Inattention	.81***	.66***	.82***
CPRS Hyperactive–Impulsive	.56***	.85***	.77***
CPRS Learning Problems	.58***	.42**	.55***
CPRS Executive Functioning	.72***	.47**	.66***
CPRS Aggression	.31*	.09	.22
CPRS Peer Relations	.23	–.01	.12
CPRS Global Index	.67***	.67***	.73***
CPRS DSM CD	.22	.03	.15
CPRS DSM ODD	.50***	.34*	.46**

Note. CPRS, Conners Parent Rating Scale; CD, conduct disorder; ODD, oppositional defiant disorder.
$^*p < .05$; $^{**}p < .01$; $^{***}p < .001$.

ranged from .01 to .85, with 28 of 36 values achieving statistical significance. If a Bonferroni correction is applied to control Type I error rate for multiple correlations (i.e., alpha = .001), 23 of these correlations can be considered statistically significant. As was the case for teacher ratings, the strongest correlations were found between factor scores on the ADHD Rating Scale–5, Home Version, and CPRS ADHD-related factor scores (i.e., DSM-Inattentive, DSM-Hyperactive–Impulsive, ADHD Index, Inattention, and Hyperactive–Impulsive). In fact, ratings of ADHD symptoms on these two measures shared between 29 and 72% of the variance. The pattern of correlations provided initial evidence for the discriminant validity of the Inattention and Hyperactivity–Impulsivity subscales. For example, the Inattention scale was more strongly related to CPRS inattention-related factors (i.e., DSM-Inattentive, Inattention) than was the Hyperactivity–Impulsivity scale. Conversely, the Hyperactivity–Impulsivity scale was more strongly related to CPRS hyperactivity–impulsivity-related factors (i.e., DSM-Hyperactive–Impulsive, Hyperactive–Impulsive) than was the Inattention scale. Furthermore, the Inattention scale was more strongly related to CPRS Executive Functioning and Learning Problems, and DSM ODD scales.

Parent ratings of ADHD symptoms were also significantly related to key areas of parent-reported functional impairment on the IRS (see Table 4.5). After correction for Type I error, Inattention scale scores were significantly related to IRS Parent–Child Conflict, Academic, and Family scores; all correlations were in the medium range. Hyperactivity–Impulsivity scale scores were significantly related to IRS Sibling Relationships, Academic, Chores, and Family; however, none of these were statistically significant after a Bonferroni correction was applied. Total score was significantly correlated with IRS Peer Relationships, Sibling Relationships, Conflict, Academic, Chores, Family, and Need for Treatment scores; with three correlations remaining statistically significant after a Bonferroni correction was applied.

TABLE 4.5. Validity Coefficients for ADHD Rating Scale–5, Home Version, Symptom Ratings with Impairment Rating Scale Scores

Measure	Inattention	Hyperactivity–Impulsivity	Total
IRS Peers	.28	.25	.32*
IRS Best Friend	–.08	–.15	–.11
IRS Siblings	.52**	.46**	.55***
IRS Conflict	.55***	.31	.48**
IRS Academic	.60***	.32*	.52***
IRS Classroom	.12	–.14	–.01
IRS Chores	.51	.74**	.70*
IRS Self-Esteem	.25	.20	.25
IRS Family	.60***	.39*	.56***
IRS Need for Treatment	.41**	.27	.40**

Note. IRS, Impairment Rating Scale.
$^*p > .05$; $^{**}p > .01$; $^{***}p > .001$.

Relationships between Teacher ADHD Impairment Ratings and Criterion Measures

Spearman rho correlations between scores on the six ADHD Rating Scale–5, School Version, impairment dimensions and teacher ratings on the IRS are displayed in Table 4.6. Spearman rho correlations were used because impairment item scores can be considered ordinal level data. The absolute value of validity coefficients ranged from .05 to .90, with 36 of 42 correlations significantly greater than 0 after Bonferroni correction for control of Type I error. Correlations were generally moderate to large in magnitude. When correlations with IRS Best Friend were excluded (as these were all small and not statistically significant), ADHD Rating Scale–5 Impairment and IRS ratings shared between 21 to 81% variance. As expected, the strongest correlations were found between ADHD Rating Scale–5 Relationships with School Professionals and IRS Teacher (r = .83); ADHD Rating Scale–5 Peers and IRS Peers (r = .80); ADHD Rating Scale–5 Homework and IRS Academic (r = .68); and ADHD Rating Scale–5 Academics and IRS Academic (r = .90). ADHD Rating Scale–5 Behavior was strongly related to IRS Peers, Self-Esteem, and Need for Treatment, while ADHD Rating Scale–5 Self-Esteem was most highly correlated with IRS Peers, Classroom, Self-Esteem, and Need for Treatment. Although the direction of obtained correlations between impairment ratings on the ADHD Rating Scale–5 and direct observations of classroom behavior and performance were in the expected direction (i.e., positive correlations with off-task behavior, negative correlations with engaged behavior and percentage correct), only a few were statistically significant (see Table 4.7). Specifically, Relationship with School Professionals was negatively correlated with percentage correct (r = –.63), Relationship with Peers was positively correlated with off-task verbal behavior (r = .43), Academics was positively correlated with off-task motor behavior (r = .49), and Self-Esteem was negatively correlated with percentage correct (r = –.55). The low number of statistically significant correlations is most likely due, in part, to the limited power afforded by our modest sample size.

TABLE 4.6. Validity Coefficients for ADHD Rating Scale–5, School Version, Impairment Ratings with Impairment Rating Scale Scores

Measure	Professionals	Peers	Homework	Academics	Behavior	Self-Esteem
IRS Peers	.66***	.80***	.52***	.60***	.71***	.75***
IRS Best Friend	.16	–.06	.05	.09	.08	.17
IRS Teacher	.83***	.46***	.57***	.65***	.60***	.55***
IRS Academic	.68***	.51***	.68***	.90***	.67***	.70***
IRS Classroom	.64***	.53***	.53***	.74***	.58***	.82***
IRS Self-Esteem	.72***	.66***	.59***	.71***	.72***	.73***
IRS Need for Treatment	.70***	.57***	.62***	.84***	.72***	.76***

Note. IRS, Impairment Rating Scale.
***p > .001.

TABLE 4.7. Validity Coefficients for ADHD Rating Scale–5, School Version, Impairment Ratings with Direct Observation and Classroom Measures

Measure	Professionals	Peers	Homework	Academics	Behavior	Self-Esteem
BOSS Active Engaged	–.09	–.03	–.13	–.19	.04	–.20
BOSS Passive Engaged	–.09	–.18	–.01	–.10	–.22	–.06
BOSS Off-Task Motor	.28	.08	.13	.49**	.25	.24
BOSS Off-Task Passive	.15	.02	.20	.35	.10	.25
BOSS Off-Task Verbal	.30	.43*	–.08	.08	.28	.31
Percentage Correct	–.63**	–.16	–.32	–.42	–.46	–.55*

Note. BOSS, Behavior Observation of Students in Schools.
$*p < .05$; $**p < .01$.

Relationships between Parent ADHD Impairment Ratings and Criterion Measures

Spearman rho correlations between scores on the six ADHD Rating Scale–5, Home Version, impairment dimensions and parent ratings on the IRS are displayed in Table 4.8. The absolute value of validity coefficients ranged from .01 to .94, with 29 of 60 correlations significantly greater than 0; 15 correlations remained significant after Bonferroni correction for control of Type I error. Correlations ranged from small to large in magnitude. ADHD Rating Scale–5 impairment and IRS ratings shared between 0 to 88% variance. As expected, the strongest correlations were found between ADHD Rating Scale–5 Family Relationships and IRS Siblings ($r = .55$) and Family ($r = .52$); ADHD Rating Scale–5 Homework and IRS Academic ($r = .80$); ADHD Rating Scale–5 Academics and IRS Academic ($r = .81$); and ADHD Rating Scale–5 Behavior and IRS Classroom ($r = .94$). Furthermore, ADHD Rating

TABLE 4.8. Validity Coefficients for ADHD Rating Scale–5, Home Version, Impairment Ratings with Impairment Rating Scale Scores

Measure	Family	Peers	Homework	Academics	Behavior	Self-Esteem
IRS Peers	.13	.40**	.34*	.08	.28	.05
IRS Best Friend	–.16	–.14	–.05	.01	–.10	.01
IRS Siblings	.55**	.34*	.63***	.66***	.46**	–.03
IRS Conflict	.47**	.36*	.72***	.63***	.34*	–.16
IRS Academic	.44**	.45**	.80***	.81***	.53***	–.10
IRS Classroom	–.09	–.14	–.18	.00	.94***	–.14
IRS Chores	.25	–.29	.47	.61*	.34	–.29
IRS Self-Esteem	.03	.20	.25	.00	.17	.15
IRS Family	.52***	.46**	.80***	.68***	.63***	–.08
IRS Need for Treatment	.44**	.42**	.67***	.63***	.34*	–.04

Note. IRS, Impairment Rating Scale.
$*p < .05$; $**p < .01$; $***p < .001$.

Scale–5 Family Relationships was significantly correlated with IRS Parent–Child Conflict, Academic, and Need for Treatment. ADHD Rating Scale–5 Relationship with Peers was significantly correlated with IRS Peers, Siblings, Parent–Child Conflict, Academics, Family, and Need for Treatment. ADHD Rating Scale–5 Homework was also significantly related with IRS Peers, Siblings, Parent–Child Conflict, Family Relationships, and Need for Treatment. ADHD Rating Scale–5 Academics was also correlated with IRS Siblings, Parent–Child Conflict, Chores, Family, and Need for Treatment. ADHD Rating Scale–5 Behavior was also correlated with IRS Siblings, Parent–Child Conflict, Academic, Family, and Need for Treatment. Scores on Self-Esteem were not significantly correlated with any IRS score.

Sample and Procedures: Discriminant Validity

Participants

The sample used to examine the discriminant validity of parent and teacher ratings on the ADHD Rating Scale–IV consisted of consecutive referrals to the ADHD Evaluation and Treatment Program of the Children's Seashore House in Philadelphia (now The Children's Hospital of Philadelphia). All children were referred for an initial evaluation or a reevaluation of ADHD. Participants met the following inclusion criteria: (1) completion by parents and teachers of the ADHD Rating Scale–IV and a diagnostic interview with parents using the Diagnostic Interview for Children and Adolescents—Revised (DICA-R; Reich, Shayka, & Taibleson, 1991) updated to reflect DSM-IV criteria (Eiraldi, Power, & Nezu, 1997); and (2) estimated IQ of 80 or above on the Kaufman Brief Intelligence Test (KBIT; Kaufman & Kaufman, 1990). Children were excluded if they presented evidence of pervasive developmental disorder, a psychotic disorder, or a progressive neurological disorder. Children were also excluded if they took a psychotropic medication for ADHD or related disorders within 6 months of the time of evaluation.

The sample consisted of 92 children (24 girls, 68 boys) between the ages of 6 and 14.75 years ($M = 9.0$, $SD = 2.2$; see Power, Doherty, et al., 1998). Grade levels ranged from kindergarten through grade 8, with 73% of the sample attending grades 1 through 4. The distribution of ethnic groups represented was 21.7% African American, 3.3% Hispanic, and 75% white. The range of socioeconomic levels as assessed by the Four Factor Index of Social Status (Hollingshead, 1975) was as follows: 3.2% in Category I (unskilled laborers), 14.2% in Category II (machine operators, semiskilled workers), 25% in Category III (skilled craftsmen, clerical, sales workers), 40.2% in Category IV (small business owners, technicians), and 17.4% in Category V (major business owners, professionals). On the KBIT, the sample achieved mean scores of 103.1 ($SD = 11.9$) on the Vocabulary scale, 100.5 ($SD = 11.7$) on Matrices, and 101.9 ($SD = 11.1$) on the Composite.

Procedures

Parents and teachers completed the Child Behavior Checklist (CBCL; Achenbach, 1991a, 1991b, 1991c), the teacher-rated Child Attention Problems scale (CAP;

Barkley, 1990), and home and school versions of the ADHD Rating Scale–IV prior to their initial clinic visit. The DICA-R was conducted by a doctoral-level psychology clinician or an advanced doctoral candidate in psychology at the initial clinic visit.

Children were assigned to a diagnostic group or clinical control group on the basis of their scores on a multimethod assessment battery including the parent version of the DICA-R, the parent-rated CBCL, and the teacher-rated CAP. Children were categorized as having ADHD, Predominantly Inattentive presentation (ADHD/I) if they demonstrated the following: (1) a DICA-R diagnosis of ADHD/I, (2) a *T* score of 60 or above on the Attention Problems factor of the CBCL, and (3) a score on the Inattention subscale of the CAP greater than or equal to the 93rd percentile. Children were diagnosed with ADHD, Combined presentation (ADHD/COM) if they demonstrated (1) a DICA-R diagnosis of ADHD/COM, (2) a *T* score of 60 or above on the Attention Problems factor of the CBCL, and (3) scores on the Inattention and Overactivity subscales of the CAP greater than or equal to the 93rd percentile. Two children met the criteria for ADHD, Predominantly Hyperactive–Impulsive presentation, and were not included in further analyses. Remaining children who did not meet the criteria for any of the ADHD presentations were assigned to a clinical control group.

Based on these criteria, 30 children were classified as having ADHD/I, 25 participants had ADHD/COM, and 35 children were assigned to the clinical control group. Although the ADHD/COM group had a higher proportion of participants with a comorbid conduct disorder, there were no further differences between groups with respect to psychiatric comorbidity, gender, age, or special education placement.

Discriminant Validity of Parent and Teacher Ratings

Means and standard deviations for parent and teacher Inattention and Hyperactivity–Impulsivity scores across three groups (ADHD/COM, ADHD/I, and clinical control) are presented in Table 4.9. Statistically significant differences in mean ratings between these three groups were obtained for parent Inattention

TABLE 4.9. Means and Standard Deviations of ADHD Rating Scale–IV Scores across Clinical Groups

	Group		
Measure	Control	ADHD/I	ADHD/COM
Parent Inattention	14.2 (7.9)[a]	19.3 (4.4)[b]	19.3 (4.3)[b]
Parent Hyperactivity–Impulsivity	11.6 (8.0)[a]	10.7 (5.7)[a]	16.4 (5.9)[b]
Teacher Inattention	13.3 (5.9)[a]	19.3 (4.7)[b]	21.6 (4.3)[b]
Teacher Hyperactivity–Impulsivity	10.5 (8.0)[a]	6.9 (4.5)[a]	18.6 (5.7)[b]

Note. ADHD/I, ADHD predominantly inattentive presentation; ADHD/COM, ADHD combined presentation. Standard deviations are in parentheses. Means with different superscripts were significantly different at the $p < .05$ level. From DuPaul, Power, McGoey, et al. (1998). Copyright 1998 by Sage Publications. Reprinted by permission.

ratings ($F(2, 87) = 7.56$, $p < .001$), parent Hyperactivity–Impulsivity ratings ($F(2, 87) = 5.60$, $p < .01$), teacher Inattention ratings ($F(2, 87) = 22.34$, $p < .0001$), and teacher Hyperactivity–Impulsivity ratings ($F(2, 87) = 23.57$, $p < .0001$). Tukey HSD post hoc comparisons (conducted using an alpha level of .05) indicated that parent and teacher Inattention ratings were significantly higher (indicating greater levels of inattention) for participants in the predominantly Inattentive and Combined presentation groups relative to clinical controls. Alternatively, parent and teacher Hyperactivity–Impulsivity ratings were significantly higher for participants in the Combined presentation group relative to their counterparts in the other two groups. There were no significant differences in parent and teacher Hyperactivity–Impulsivity scores between the predominantly Inattentive presentation and clinical control participants.

Predictive Validity

To further evaluate the validity of the ADHD Rating Scale–IV, we investigated the ability of this measure to differentiate children with ADHD from those without this disorder as well as to distinguish children with the two most common presentations of ADHD, the Combined presentation (ADHD/COM) and the Inattentive presentation (ADHD/I). We conducted predictive validity studies in both a clinical and a school setting.

Prediction in a Clinical Setting

The sample and procedures for diagnosing participants in our clinic-based predictive validity study (see Power, Doherty, et al., 1998) were described in the previous section under "Sample and Procedures: Discriminant Validity."

Logistic regression methods were used to evaluate (1) whether parent and teacher ratings used separately were able to differentiate clinical groups from the control group, and clinical groups from each other, and (2) whether a strategy combining parent and teacher ratings achieved a higher level of diagnostic accuracy than a single-informant approach. Logistic regression generates a correlation-type statistic (R) reflecting the unique association between each predictor variable and the criterion variable (i.e., diagnostic group membership), and a chi-square statistic indicating whether the logistic model results in a significant level of prediction and whether each additional variable entered into the model results in an improvement in prediction.

Predictive Validity of the Inattention Subscale

Table 4.10 presents the results of logistic regression analyses evaluating the ability of the Inattention subscale to differentiate children with ADHD/I from those in the control group. Both teacher ratings and parent ratings, when entered separately, were predictive of membership in the ADHD/I versus control group. The association between teacher ratings of Inattention and diagnostic status was moderate ($R = .38$), and the association between parent ratings of Inattention and diagnostic status was low ($R = .26$). In a forward stepwise logistic regression analysis, teacher ratings entered the equation first. The addition of parent ratings resulted in a significant improvement of the logistic model (χ^2 (1) = 6.85, $p < .01$). The combination of teacher and parent ratings in the model correctly classified 72% of the cases; however, this was slightly less than the percentage predicted by teacher ratings alone (74%).

Next, logistic regression analyses were used to evaluate the ability of the Inattention subscale to differentiate children with ADHD/COM from those in the control group (see Table 4.10). Once again, both teacher ratings and parent ratings, when entered separately, were predictive of membership in the ADHD/COM group versus the control group. The association between teacher ratings of Inattention and diagnostic status was moderate ($R = .44$). The use of teacher ratings alone correctly classified 80% of the participants. In contrast, the association between parent ratings of Inattention and diagnostic status was low ($R = .23$). In a forward stepwise logistic regression analysis, teacher ratings entered the equation first; the addition of parent ratings did not result in a significant improvement of the logistic model.

Predictive Validity of the Hyperactivity–Impulsivity Subscale

Table 4.11 presents the results of logistic regression analyses used to evaluate the ability of the Hyperactivity–Impulsivity subscale to differentiate children with ADHD/COM from those in the control group. Both teacher and parent ratings, when entered separately, were able to predict membership in the ADHD/COM versus control group. The association between teacher ratings of Hyperactivity–Impulsivity and diagnostic status was low to moderate ($R = .32$), and the association between parent ratings of Hyperactivity–Impulsivity and diagnostic status was low ($R = .22$). In a forward stepwise logistic regression analysis, teacher ratings entered the equation first. The addition of parent ratings resulted in significant improvement of the logistic model (χ^2 (1) = 7.18, $p < .01$). The combination of teacher and parent ratings in the model correctly classified 75% of the cases.

Next, logistic regression analyses were used to evaluate the ability of the Hyperactivity–Impulsivity subscale to differentiate children with ADHD/COM from those with ADHD/I (see Table 4.11). Both teacher and parent ratings,

TABLE 4.10. Results of Logistic Regression Analyses When Using the Inattention Subscale: Clinic-Based Study

Comparison	χ^2	p	R	Prediction
ADHD/I versus control group				
Teacher ratings	18.68	.0001	.38	74%
Parent ratings	10.72	.0001	.26	68%
ADHD/COM versus control group				
Teacher ratings	24.11	.0001	.44	80%
Parent ratings	8.08	.005	.23	62%

TABLE 4.11. Results of Logistic Regression Analyses When Using the Hyperactivity–Impulsivity Subscale: Clinic-Based Study

Comparison	χ^2	p	R	Prediction
ADHD/COM versus control group				
Teacher ratings	12.70	.001	.32	65%
Parent ratings	6.95	.01	.22	60%
ADHD/COM versus ADHD/I				
Teacher ratings	30.14	.0001	.46	84%
Parent ratings	7.69	.01	.24	64%

when entered separately, were able to predict membership in the ADHD/COM group versus the ADHD/I group. The association between teacher ratings of Hyperactivity–Impulsivity and diagnostic status was moderate (R = .46); teacher ratings correctly classified 84% of the cases. In contrast, the association between parent ratings of Hyperactivity–Impulsivity and diagnostic status was low (R = .24). In a forward stepwise logistic regression analysis, teacher ratings only entered the equation first; the addition of parent ratings failed to result in significant improvement of the logistic model.

Conclusions

Results from the clinic-based study demonstrated that the Inattention subscale was able to differentiate children with ADHD/I from a control group, and children with ADHD/COM from controls. In addition, logistic regression analyses indicated that the Hyperactivity–Impulsivity subscale successfully differentiated children with ADHD/COM from controls, and children with ADHD/COM from those with ADHD/I. The results revealed that teacher ratings on the ADHD Rating Scale–IV are extremely important in predicting ADHD presentation status. Although parent ratings were also significantly predictive of diagnostic status, teacher ratings were better at predicting ADHD presentation status than parent ratings. Furthermore, the results suggested that an approach to diagnostic prediction that includes both teachers and parents is often superior to a single-informant approach.

Prediction in a School Setting

Participants in our school-based predictive validity study (see Power, Andrews, et al., 1998) were referred students from two school districts, both of which served children in kindergarten through eighth grade. Participants were students in general education referred by their teachers to the school's Pupil Assistance Committee (PAC) for academic and/or behavioral problems. During the course of the study, 259 students were referred to PAC teams. Parents of students referred to PAC received a letter informing them about the study and requesting permission for their child to be screened for attention and behavior problems through the use of parent and teacher rating scales. One hundred fifty-six (60%) of the parents or guardians gave permission for their child to be screened. Nine students were excluded because they were taking medication, leaving 147 participants, 48 of whom were girls. Students ranged in age from 5 through 14 years, with a mean of 9 years. The ethnic groups represented were 29.6% African American, 3.7% Hispanic, 1.2% Native American, 2.5% Asian American, and 61.7% white. Almost 90% of the sample was in the middle categories of socioeconomic status.

A multigate screening process was used to determine which students met the criteria for ADHD. The parents of all students referred to PAC during the course of the study were sent a letter inviting them to participate in a screening to assess attention and behavior problems. Parents who gave consent were asked to complete the ADHD Rating Scale–IV for their referred child. In addition, students whose parents granted consent were rated by teachers on the Child Attention Profile (CAP) and ADHD Rating Scale–IV. Students rated at or above the 93rd percentile on the Inattention and/or Overactivity factor of the CAP met screening criteria for ADHD and were advanced to the next stage of evaluation. Students who did not meet screening criteria were not assessed further. Ninety-five students (64.6%) met screening criteria.

For each student meeting screening criteria, parents were contacted to arrange a time for the diagnostic interview. We obtained informed consent and conducted a diagnostic interview with the parents of 76 students (80.0% of those who screened positively for ADHD). In each of these latter cases, the teacher completed the CAP a second time (CAP-2). Children were assigned to a diagnostic group or clinical control group on the basis of their scores on a multimethod assessment battery including the parent version of the DICA-R and the teacher-rated CAP-2. The ADHD Rating Scale–IV was not used to determine clinical group membership.

Children were categorized as having ADHD (any presentation) if they met criteria for any of the ADHD presentations on the DICA-R and were rated by teachers as greater than or equal to the 93rd percentile on the Inattention and/or Overactivity subscale of the CAP-2. Using these criteria, 52 children were classified as having ADHD. Presentation status was determined by the DICA-R; 29 students were diagnosed with ADHD/I, 0 with ADHD/HI, and 23 with ADHD/COM. In the sample, 76 students, including the 52 children not meeting initial screening criteria on the CAP, did not meet criteria for ADHD and were assigned to the control group. An additional 19 students met screening criteria through the use of the CAP, but we were not able to arrange a diagnostic interview with their parents.

Predictive Validity of the Inattention Subscale

Table 4.12 presents the results of logistic regression analyses used to evaluate the ability of the Inattention subscale of the ADHD Rating Scale–IV to differentiate children with ADHD/I from those in the control group. Both teacher and parent ratings, when entered separately, predicted membership in the ADHD/I group versus the control group. The association between teacher ratings of Inattention and diagnostic status was low to moderate (R = .32), as was the association between parent ratings of Inattention and diagnostic status (R = .27). In a forward stepwise logistic regression analysis, teacher ratings entered the equation first. The addition of parent ratings resulted in a significant improvement of the logistic model (χ^2 (1) = 7.90, $p < .01$). The combination of teacher and parent ratings in the model correctly classified 78% of the cases.

Next, logistic regression analyses were used to evaluate the ability of the Inattention subscale to differentiate children with ADHD/COM from those in the control group (see Table 4.12). Both teacher and parent ratings, when entered separately, predicted membership in the ADHD/COM group versus the control group. The association between teacher ratings of Inattention and diagnostic status was low to moderate (R = .36), as was the association between parent ratings of Inattention and diagnostic status (R = .36). In a forward stepwise logistic regression analysis, teacher ratings entered the equation first; the addition of parent ratings resulted in a significant improvement of the logistic model (χ^2 (1) = 12.29, $p < .001$). The combination of teacher and parent ratings in the model correctly classified 83% of the cases.

Predictive Validity of the Hyperactivity–Impulsivity Subscale

Logistic regression analyses were used to evaluate the ability of the Hyperactivity–Impulsivity subscale to differentiate children with ADHD/COM from those in the control group (see Table 4.13). Both teacher and parent ratings, when entered separately, were able to predict membership in the ADHD/COM group versus the control group. The association between teacher ratings of Hyperactivity–Impulsivity and diagnostic status was low (R = .26), but the association between parent ratings of Hyperactivity–Impulsivity and diagnostic status was moderate (R = .40). In a forward stepwise logistic regression analysis, parent ratings entered the equation first. The addition of teacher ratings resulted in significant improvement of the logistic model (χ^2 (1) = 6.04, $p < .05$). The combination of teacher and parent ratings in the model correctly classified 83% of the cases.

Next, logistic regression analyses were used to evaluate the ability of the Hyperactivity–Impulsivity subscale to differentiate children with ADHD/COM from those with ADHD/I (see Table 4.13). When teacher ratings were entered alone in the analysis, the resultant model was not able to differentiate children with

TABLE 4.12. Results of Logistic Regression Analyses When Using the Inattention Subscale: School-Based Study

Comparison	χ^2	p	R	Prediction
ADHD/I versus control group				
Teacher ratings	15.65	.0001	.32	75%
Parent ratings	11.52	.001	.27	76%
ADHD/COM versus control group				
Teacher ratings	18.15	.0001	.36	78%
Parent ratings	20.30	.0001	.36	80%

TABLE 4.13. Results of Logistic Regression Analyses When Using the Hyperactivity–Impulsivity Subscale: School-Based Study

Comparison	χ^2	p	R	Prediction
ADHD/COM versus control group				
Teacher ratings	9.88	.01	.26	78%
Parent ratings	22.51	.0001	.40	82%
ADHD/COM versus ADHD/I				
Teacher ratings	2.66	n.s.	.08	62%
Parent ratings	17.46	.0001	.39	79%

ADHD/COM from those with ADHD/I at a statistically significant level. Alternatively, parent ratings, when entered alone, were able to differentiate ADHD/COM from ADHD/I and correctly classified 79% of the cases. The association between parent ratings of Hyperactivity–Impulsivity and diagnostic status was moderate (R = .39). In a forward stepwise logistic regression analysis, parent ratings only entered the equation first; the addition of teacher ratings did not result in a significant improvement of the logistic model.

Conclusions

The results of the school-based study indicated that the Inattention and Hyperactivity–Impulsivity subscales of the ADHD Rating Scale–IV succeeded in predicting group membership in the ADHD/COM and ADHD/I groups. Logistic regression analyses revealed that the Inattention subscale was accurate in differentiating children with ADHD/I and ADHD/COM from the control group. Moreover, logistic regression analyses showed that the Hyperactivity–Impulsivity subscale successfully differentiated children with ADHD/COM from controls, as well as children with ADHD/COM from those with ADHD/I. The pattern of results differed somewhat, depending on whether the Inattention subscale or the Hyperactivity–Impulsivity subscale was being used for prediction. When predictions were based on the Inattention subscale, both teachers and parents made a significant and essentially equal contribution to the prediction of diagnostic status. This finding was demonstrated in the prediction of children with ADHD/I, as well as in the prediction of those with ADHD/COM. Even though teacher ratings entered the equation first in a forward stepwise analysis, parent ratings made an additional significant contribution to the prediction of diagnostic status.

In making predictions based on ratings on the Hyperactivity–Impulsivity subscale, parent ratings in general were more accurate than teacher ratings. Both teacher and parent ratings of Hyperactivity–Impulsivity made a significant contribution to the prediction of children with ADHD/COM versus those in the control group, but parent ratings clearly made a stronger contribution to prediction. Further, parent ratings, but not teacher ratings, of Hyperactivity–Impulsivity were successful in differentiating between the two presentations of ADHD.

Summary and Conclusions

Our analyses indicate that the Home and School Versions of the ADHD Rating Scale–5 have adequate psychometric properties for use as screening, diagnostic, and treatment outcome measures. As was found for the prior version of the ADHD Rating Scale (DuPaul, Power, McGoey, Ikeda, & Anastopoulos, 1998), subscales on both versions of the rating scale were found to have high levels of internal consistency and test–retest reliability. Teacher ratings were found to have greater stability over time than parent ratings, particularly for inattention symptoms and for youth in the younger age group (5–10 years). This result affirms the importance of obtaining teacher ratings as part of a comprehensive diagnostic assessment of ADHD. The lower stability of parent ratings in the adolescent group (11–17 years) may reflect a decline in parental surveillance of youth activities with increasing age. Furthermore, symptom subscale scores were found to correlate significantly with questionnaires assessing ADHD symptoms (Conners Parent and Teacher Rating Scales) and symptom-related impairment (Impairment Rating Scale). Parent and teacher ratings of symptom-related impairment correlated with similar functional impairment items on the IRS with stronger validity coefficients found for teacher impairment ratings relative to parent impairment ratings. Teacher ratings of ADHD symptoms were found to correlate significantly with observed classroom off-task behavior, while teacher ratings of symptom-related impairment were correlated with off-task behavior and academic performance (i.e., accuracy of student academic work samples). Parent and teacher ratings on the previous version of the ADHD Rating Scale (i.e., ADHD Rating Scale–IV) were demonstrated to discriminate between children representing different ADHD presentations (i.e., Combined vs. Predominantly Inattentive), as well as between children with ADHD and clinic-referred children who did not have ADHD. Finally, the combination of parent and teacher ratings was found to predict diagnosis of ADHD in the context of both clinic-based and school-based assessments. When used as part of a comprehensive assessment battery that includes diagnostic interviews, behavior observations, and related measures, the ADHD Rating Scale–5 can provide reliable and valid data regarding the frequency of ADHD symptoms and severity of ADHD symptom-related impairment.

CHAPTER 5

Interpretation and Use of the Scales for Diagnostic and Screening Purposes

In selecting a rating scale for assessing ADHD, it is not sufficient to know that the measure has acceptable psychometric properties. A clinician must also know how useful the measure is in diagnosing ADHD and screening out children and adolescents who do not have this disorder. To evaluate the clinical utility of an instrument, it is important to examine its sensitivity and specificity as well as its positive predictive power (PPP) and negative predictive power (NPP). This chapter describes research we conducted to evaluate the clinical utility of the ADHD Rating Scale–5 in a parent-referred clinical setting and a teacher-referred school setting. Some of this work was conducted with the previous version of our scale (i.e., the ADHD Rating Scale–IV; DuPaul, Power, et al., 1998). Although the symptom items of the ADHD Rating Scale–5 correspond closely with those of the ADHD Rating Scale–IV, particularly for children between the ages of 5 and 10 years, clinicians should exercise some caution in applying recommended cutoff points when using the current version for screening or diagnosing ADHD. This chapter concludes by describing brief case studies to illustrate how to use this scale in clinical decision making.

Diagnosing ADHD

Specificity and PPP are especially helpful statistics for determining the degree to which a measure is useful in diagnosing or "ruling in" a disorder. Specificity, as it pertains to the use of rating scales, refers to the probability that children known to not have a disorder are rated below a particular cutoff score. For instance, if the specificity associated with a score at the 93rd percentile on a measure of

Inattention is .90, this means that 90% of children without ADHD will score below this cutoff point. Specificity reflects the confidence one has in generalizing from a disorder to a behavior or score, which is a deductive process. In contrast, PPP refers to the probability that a child has a disorder, given the presence of a score at or above a designated cutoff point on a diagnostic measure. For instance, if the PPP associated with a score at the 93rd percentile on a measure of Inattention is .90, this means that 90% of children scoring at or above this cutoff point have ADHD. Thus PPP represents the confidence a clinician can have in generalizing from a score to a disorder, which is the inductive process typically used in clinical decision making. Sensitivity is also a useful statistic in determining the optimal cutoff point on a scale. Sensitivity refers to the probability that children known to have a disorder are rated at or above a particular cutoff score. For instance, if the sensitivity associated with a score at the 93rd percentile on a measure of Inattention is .90, this means that 90% of children with ADHD will score at or above this cutoff point. A consideration of sensitivity is important in order to maximize the percentage of cases with ADHD that get accurately detected by the scale.

Screening for ADHD

Sensitivity and NPP are especially helpful in determining the degree to which a measure is useful in screening to rule out a disorder. Sensitivity is crucial for screening because it is important to ensure that a high percentage of cases with ADHD score above the cutoff point and do not get screened out. NPP refers to the probability that a child does not have a disorder given a score below a designated cutoff point on a diagnostic measure. For instance, if the NPP associated with a score at the 85th percentile on a measure of Inattention is .90, this means that 90% of children scoring below this cutoff score do not have ADHD. Like PPP, NPP represents the confidence a clinician can have in generalizing from a behavior or score to a disorder. Specificity is also important to consider when determining the optimal cutoff point for screening in order to maximize the number of cases without ADHD that get eliminated through the screening process, thereby minimizing the resources needed for more expensive diagnostic evaluation.

Several researchers have argued that in evaluating the clinical utility of a measure, PPP and NPP are more important than sensitivity and specificity (Chen, Faraone, Biederman, & Tsuang, 1994; Laurent, Landau, & Stark, 1993). In fact, both sets of constructs are important to consider in determining the utility of a measure and the optimal choice of cutoff scores (Power & Bradley-Klug, 2013), as is illustrated in this chapter.

Selecting the Optimal Cutoff Score

The choice of an optimal cutoff score on a scale varies, depending on the purpose of an assessment. If an examiner is performing a screening of ADHD in the general population of children, it is important to select a cutoff score that is highly accurate in predicting the absence of ADHD (NPP), as well as one that is able to detect a relatively high percentage of children who have ADHD (sensitivity) while still eliminating a reasonably high percentage of children without the disorder (specificity). For screening, it is generally preferable to err on the side of being *inclusive* of children with ADHD, as opposed to exclusive of these youngsters, knowing that a more comprehensive evaluation conducted at a later time will provide more conclusive diagnostic information. Furthermore, when an examiner performs a diagnostic assessment, selection of a cutoff score that is highly accurate in predicting the presence of ADHD (PPP), as well as one that is able to exclude a relatively high percentage of children who do not have ADHD (specificity) while including a reasonably high percentage who have the disorder (sensitivity), is critical. For the purposes of diagnostic assessment, it is preferable to err on the side of being *exclusive*. Given that the diagnosis of ADHD often has implications for medication use and school decision making and programming, it is important for the examiner to be quite certain of an accurate diagnosis and to identify few false positives.

Research on the Clinical Utility of the ADHD Rating Scale–IV

We conducted two studies, a clinic-based and a school-based study, to evaluate the clinical utility of the ADHD Rating Scale–IV (Power, Andrews, et al., 1998; Power, Doherty, et al., 1998) using symptom severity ratings. The methodology for these studies is described in Chapter 4 in the sections on discriminant and predictive validity. For both the clinic-based sample and school-based sample, symptom utility estimates (sensitivity, specificity, PPP, and NPP) were used to determine optimal cutoff scores on the Inattention subscale of the ADHD Rating Scale–IV for differentiating (1) children with ADHD/I from a clinical control group without any subtype of ADHD and (2) children with ADHD/COM from clinical controls. Symptom utility estimates were also used to determine the optimal cutoff scores on the Hyperactivity–Impulsivity subscale for differentiating (1) children with ADHD/COM from clinical controls and (2) children with ADHD/I from those with ADHD/COM.

A problem with using PPP and NPP is that these statistics are highly sensitive to base rates of symptoms (cutoffs) and diagnoses in a sample (Verhulst & Koot, 1992). Thus to make comparisons about the clinical utility of one cutoff score versus another, each of which may have a different base rate in the sample, it is necessary to employ a kappa statistic that corrects for the number of accurate predictions based on chance alone. Formulas for the kappa statistics used in our study to correct PPP (cPPP) and NPP (cNPP) are reported in Frick and colleagues (1994).

Prediction in a Clinic-Based Setting

Clinical Utility of the Inattention Subscale in a Clinic Setting

Children in the age range from 6 to 14 years participated in the clinic-based study. Symptom utility estimates associated with a series of possible cutoff scores on the Inattention subscale of the ADHD Rating Scale–IV, as rated by teachers and parents separately, are provided in Table 5.1. This table indicates base rates, sensitivity, specificity, PPP, cPPP, NPP, and cNPP statistics associated with each cutoff score (80th, 85th, 90th, 93rd, and 98th percentiles) investigated in the clinic-based study described in Chapter 4. Table 5.1 presents data regarding the ability of the Inattention subscale, as rated by teachers and parents, to differentiate children with ADHD/I from controls, as well as to differentiate children with ADHD/COM from the control group. The strategy for determining optimal thresholds was to identify the cutoff score associated with the highest level of accurate prediction (cPPP or cNPP) that resulted in a reasonable level of sensitivity or specificity. For purposes of this study, a cutoff score generally was considered clinically useful if cPPP or cNPP was greater than or equal to .65 and sensitivity or specificity was approximately .50 or greater.

TABLE 5.1 Symptom Utility Estimates Associated with Cutoff Scores on the Inattention Subscale: Clinic-Based Study

Cutoff score	Base rate	Sensitivity	Specificity	PPP (cPPP)	NPP (cNPP)
		Differentiating ADHD/I from controls—Teacher ratings			
≥ 98	.11	.20	.97	.85 (.73)	.59 (.10)
≥ 93	.37	.63	.86	.79 (.61)	.73 (.42)
≥ 90	.42	.67	.80	.74 (.52)	.74 (.43)
≥ 85	.54	.77	.66	.66 (.36)	.77 (.49)
≥ 80	.71	.90	.46	.59 (.23)	.84 (.66)
		Differentiating ADHD/COM from controls—Teacher ratings			
≥ 98	.10	.20	.97	.83 (.71)	.63 (.11)
≥ 93	.38	.72	.86	.78 (.63)	.81 (.54)
≥ 90	.45	.80	.80	.74 (.56)	.85 (.64)
≥ 85	.55	.84	.66	.64 (.38)	.85 (.64)
≥ 80	.70	.92	.46	.55 (.22)	.89 (.73)
		Differentiating ADHD/I from controls—Parent ratings			
≥ 98	.35	.47	.74	.61 (.27)	.62 (.17)
≥ 93	.66	.83	.49	.58 (.22)	.77 (.51)
≥ 90	.75	.93	.40	.57 (.20)	.88 (.73)
≥ 85	.77	.93	.37	.56 (.18)	.87 (.71)
≥ 80	.83	.93	.26	.52 (.11)	.82 (.61)
		Differentiating ADHD/COM from controls—Parent ratings			
≥ 98	.27	.28	.74	.44 (.04)	.59 (.02)
≥ 93	.65	.84	.49	.54 (.21)	.81 (.54)
≥ 90	.73	.92	.40	.52 (.18)	.88 (.70)
≥ 85	.77	.96	.37	.52 (.18)	.93 (.83)
≥ 80	.85	1 .00	.26	.49 (.13)	1.00 (1.00)

Note. Cutoff scores are percentile values. Base rate refers to the proportion of children in the clinical and control groups scoring at or above the specified cutoff score. PPP refers to positive predictive power and NPP refers to negative predictive power; cPPP and cNPP are kappa statistics used to correct PPP and NPP. From Power, Doherty, et al. (1998). Copyright 1998 by Plenum Publishing Corporation. Reprinted with permission from Springer Science + Business Media.

Prediction Based on a Single Informant

The optimal cutoff score for differentiating children with ADHD/I from controls, using teacher ratings on the Inattention subscale, was the 98th percentile, but this was only marginally useful: 85% of the children scoring at or above this cutoff point had ADHD/I (cPPP = .73) and 97% of children scoring below this level did not have ADHD (specificity), but only 20% of children with ADHD/I scored at or above this level (sensitivity). The optimal cutoff score on the teacher-rated Inattention subscale for ruling out ADHD/I (80th percentile) was reasonably useful; 84% of children scoring below this cutoff point did not have ADHD/I (cNPP = .66) and 92% of children scoring above this level had ADHD (sensitivity). Nonetheless, 46% of children who did not have ADHD/I scored below this cutoff point (specificity).

Teacher ratings on the Inattention subscale were also marginally useful in predicting children who had ADHD/COM. The optimal cutoff score for ruling in ADHD/COM was the 98th percentile; the optimal cutoff for ruling out this ADHD presentation was the 80th percentile. As was the case when teacher ratings were used to differentiate ADHD/I from controls, cPPP and cNPP values were relatively high, but sensitivity was quite low for diagnostic purposes and specificity was marginal for screening purposes.

Parent ratings of Inattention were not useful in predicting or ruling in a diagnosis of ADHD/I or ADHD/COM. For ruling out ADHD/I, the 90th percentile was most useful: cNPP was relatively high (.73) and sensitivity was .93, but only 40% of children without ADHD/I scored below this cutoff point. For ruling out ADHD/COM, the 85th percentile had the most utility: cNPP was high (.83) and sensitivity was .96, but only 37% of children without ADHD/COM scored below this cutoff point.

Prediction Based on Multiple Informants

Given that the results of logistic regression analyses demonstrated that the integration of teacher and parent ratings on the Inattention subscale was better than single-informant cutoff scores in predicting group membership (see Chapter 4), at least for children who met criteria for ADHD/I, symptom utility estimates for all possible combinations of parent and teacher ratings were computed. The combination cutoff scores for the Inattention subscale that had the highest level of utility for predicting ADHD/I and ADHD/COM are presented in Table 5.2. In general, the combination cutoff scores were better than the single-scale thresholds in predicting or "ruling in" ADHD/I and ADHD/COM. For example, teacher ratings greater than or equal to the 90th percentile on the Inattention subscale were associated with a diagnosis of ADHD/I in 74% of cases (cPPP = .52). However, when teacher ratings greater than or equal to the 90th percentile were combined with parent ratings greater than or equal to the 93rd percentile, the rate of prediction improved to 85% (cPPP = .72), specificity was high (.91), and sensitivity was still reasonably high (.57). The combination of parent and teacher ratings of Inattention was marginally useful in ruling out a diagnosis of ADHD/I; with teacher ratings below the 80th percentile and parent ratings below the 85th percentile, cNPP was moderate (.63), sensitivity was relatively high (.83), and specificity was .69.

TABLE 5.2. Symptom Utility Estimates Associated with the Combination of Teacher (T) and Parent (P) Ratings on the Inattention Subscale: Clinic-Based Study

Cutoff score	Base rate	Sensitivity	Specificity	PPP (cPPP)	NPP (cNPP)
		Differentiating ADHD/I from controls			
T ≥ 80, P ≥ 80	.60	.83	.60	.64 (.33)	.81 (.58)
T ≥ 80, P ≥ 85	.55	.83	.69	.69 (.43)	.83 (.63)
T ≥ 80, P ≥ 90	.55	.83	.69	.69 (.43)	.83 (.63)
T ≥ 80, P ≥ 93	.49	.77	.74	.72 (.48)	.79 (.54)
T ≥ 80, P ≥ 98	.29	.43	.82	.68 (.41)	.63 (.20)
T ≥ 85, P ≥ 80	.46	.70	.74	.70 (.44)	.74 (.44)
T ≥ 85, P ≥ 85	.43	.70	.80	.75 (.54)	.76 (.47)
T ≥ 85, P ≥ 90	.43	.70	.80	.75 (.54)	.76 (.47)
T ≥ 85, P ≥ 93	.38	.67	.86	.80 (.63)	.75 (.46)
T ≥ 85, P ≥ 98	.23	.37	.89	.73 (.50)	.62 (.18)
T ≥ 90, P ≥ 80	.37	.60	.83	.75 (.54)	.71 (.37)
T ≥ 90, P ≥ 85	.35	.60	.86	.78 (.60)	.71 (.38)
T ≥ 90, P ≥ 90	.35	.60	.86	.78 (.60)	.71 (.38)
T ≥ 90, P ≥ 93	.31	.57	.91	.85 (.72)	.62 (.18)
T ≥ 90, P ≥ 98	.18	.33	.94	.83 (.69)	.62 (.18)
		Differentiating ADHD/COM from controls			
T ≥ 80, P ≥ 80	.62	.92	.60	.62 (.35)	.91 (.79)
T ≥ 80, P ≥ 85	.55	.88	.69	.67 (.43)	.89 (.73)
T ≥ 80, P ≥ 90	.53	.84	.69	.66 (.41)	.86 (.66)
T ≥ 80, P ≥ 93	.50	.84	.74	.70 (.49)	.87 (.68)
T ≥ 80, P ≥ 98	.22	.28	.83	.54 (.21)	.62 (.08)
T ≥ 85, P ≥ 80	.50	.84	.74	.70 (.49)	.87 (.68)
T ≥ 85, P ≥ 85	.47	.84	.80	.75 (.57)	.88 (.70)
T ≥ 85, P ≥ 90	.45	.80	.80	.74 (.56)	.85 (.64)
T ≥ 85, P ≥ 93	.42	.80	.86	.80 (.66)	.86 (.66)
T ≥ 85, P ≥ 98	.17	.24	.89	.60 (.31)	.62 (.09)
T ≥ 90, P ≥ 80	.43	.80	.83	.77 (.60)	.85 (.65)
T ≥ 90, P ≥ 85	.42	.80	.86	.80 (.66)	.86 (.66)
T ≥ 90, P ≥ 90	.40	.76	.86	.79 (.64)	.83 (.60)
T ≥ 90, P ≥ 93	.37	.76	.91	.86 (.77)	.84 (.62)
T ≥ 90, P ≥ 98	.13	.24	.94	.75 (.57)	.63 (.12)

Note. From Power, Doherty, et al. (1998). Copyright 1998 by Plenum Publishing Corporation. Reprinted with permission from Springer Science + Business Media.

In regard to differentiating children with ADHD/COM from controls, combination cutoff scores involving teacher ratings at or above the 90th percentile and parent ratings at or above the 93rd percentile once again constituted the optimal combination. For instance, this combination resulted in a high level of cPPP (.77) and specificity (.91), and a reasonably high level of sensitivity (.76). For ruling out ADHD/COM, teacher ratings below the 80th percentile and parent ratings below the 85th percentile had a high degree of utility: cNPP was .73, sensitivity was .88, and 69% of children without ADHD/COM scored below these levels.

Clinical Utility of the Hyperactivity–Impulsivity Subscale in a Clinic Setting

Symptom utility estimates associated with a series of possible cutoff scores on the Hyperactivity–Impulsivity subscale of the ADHD Rating Scale–5, as rated by teachers and parents separately, are provided in Table 5.3. This table presents data regarding the ability of the Hyperactivity–Impulsivity subscale to differentiate children with ADHD/COM from controls, as well as to differentiate children with ADHD/COM from those with ADHD/I.

Prediction Based on a Single Informant

Teacher ratings of Hyperactivity–Impulsivity generally were not useful in predicting children who had ADHD/COM when this presentation was compared to

TABLE 5.3. Symptom Utility Estimates Associated with Cutoff Scores on the Hyperactivity–Impulsivity Subscale: Clinic-Based Study

Cutoff score	Base rate	Sensitivity	Specificity	PPP (cPPP)	NPP (cNPP)
		Differentiating ADHD/COM from controls—Teacher ratings			
≥ 98	.33	.48	.77	.60 (.31)	.68 (.22)
≥ 93	.47	.64	.66	.57 (.27)	.72 (.33)
≥ 90	.60	.88	.60	.61 (.33)	.88 (.70)
≥ 85	.67	.92	.51	.58 (.27)	.90 (.76)
≥ 80	.80	.96	.31	.50 (.14)	.92 (.80)
		Differentiating ADHD/COM from ADHD/I—Teacher ratings			
≥ 98	.24	.48	.97	.92 (.86)	.69 (.32)
≥ 93	.35	.64	.90	.84 (.71)	.75 (.45)
≥ 90	.51	.88	.80	.79 (.61)	.89 (.76)
≥ 85	.60	.92	.67	.70 (.44)	.91 (.80)
≥ 80	.73	.96	.47	.60 (.27)	.93 (.85)
		Differentiating ADHD/COM from controls—Parent ratings			
≥ 98	.45	.16	.63	.27 (–.34)	.47 (–.15)
≥ 93	.67	.53	.46	.46 (–.01)	.47 (–.01)
≥ 90	.68	.60	.43	.47 (.02)	.56 (.04)
≥ 85	.73	.67	.40	.49 (.05)	.58 (.10)
≥ 80	.78	.73	.26	.48 (.31)	.58 (.09)
		Differentiating ADHD/COM from ADHD/I—Parent ratings			
≥ 98	.35	.56	.83	.74 (.52)	.69 (.33)
≥ 93	.67	.84	.47	.57 (.21)	.78 (.51)
≥ 90	.71	.84	.40	.54 (.15)	.75 (.45)
≥ 85	.78	.92	.33	.53 (.15)	.83 (.63)
≥ 80	.82	.92	.27	.51 (.10)	.80 (.56)

Note. From Power, Doherty, et al. (1998). Copyright 1998 by Plenum Publishing Corporation. Reprinted with permission from Springer Science + Business Media.

controls; however, this scale was useful in ruling out a diagnosis of ADHD/COM. For instance, 90% of the children with teacher ratings below the 85th percentile did not have ADHD/COM (cNPP = .76) and sensitivity was high (.92), but specificity was marginal (.51). Parent ratings of Hyperactivity–Impulsivity were not useful in ruling in or ruling out ADHD/COM.

Teacher ratings on the Hyperactivity–Impulsivity subscale were much more useful in differentiating children with ADHD/COM from those with ADHD/I. The optimal cutoff score for predicting or ruling in ADHD/COM was judged to be the 93rd percentile: 84% of children scored at or above this level had ADHD/COM (cPPP = .71), specificity was high (.90), and sensitivity was reasonably high (.64). The Hyperactivity–Impulsivity subscale was also useful in ruling out ADHD/COM when children with the two presentations of ADHD were compared. For instance, teacher ratings below the 85th percentile resulted in a cNPP of .80, a sensitivity of .92, and a specificity of .67. Parent ratings of Hyperactivity–Impulsivity were not useful in ruling in or ruling out a diagnosis of ADHD/COM when children with these two presentations of ADHD were compared and when children with ADHD/COM were compared to controls.

Prediction Based on Multiple Informants

Given that the results of logistic regression analyses demonstrated that the integration of teacher and parent ratings on the Hyperactivity–Impulsivity subscale was better than single-informant cutoff scores in predicting children who met criteria for ADHD/COM, at least when children with ADHD/COM were contrasted with the control group (see Chapter 4), symptom utility estimates for all possible combinations of parent and teacher ratings were computed. The combination cutoff scores with the most utility are presented in Table 5.4. As expected, based on the results of logistic regression analyses, the combination cutoff scores were better than teacher ratings alone in differentiating children with ADHD/COM from the control group, but not in differentiating children with ADHD/COM from those with ADHD/I. When the ADHD/COM group was compared with the control group, the optimal combination was judged to be teacher ratings at or above the 90th percentile and parent ratings at or above the 93rd percentile; cPPP was marginal (.57) but specificity (.81) and sensitivity (.72) were reasonably high. For ruling out ADHD/COM, both when the ADHD/COM group was compared with the control group and when the ADHD/COM group was compared with the ADHD/I group, the combination cutoff scores were not as accurate as teacher ratings alone.

Conclusions: Prediction in a Clinic Setting

Optimal cutoff scores for diagnosing and ruling out ADHD in our parent-referred, clinic-based sample are summarized in Table 5.5. The optimal approach for using the Inattention subscale to diagnose ADHD/I and ADHD/COM was one that combined teacher and parent ratings. The most useful combination appeared to be teacher ratings at or above the 90th percentile and parent ratings at or above the 93rd percentile. The optimal approach to using the Inattention subscale to screen for or rule out ADHD was also a multi-informant one: Teacher ratings less

TABLE 5.4. Symptom Utility Estimates Associated with the Combination of Teacher (T) and Parent (P) Ratings on the Hyperactivity–Impulsivity Subscale: Clinic-Based Study

Cutoff score	Base rate	Sensitivity	Specificity	PPP (cPPP)	NPP (cNPP)
		Differentiating ADHD/COM from controls			
T ≥ 80, P ≥ 80	.63	.88	.54	.58 (.28)	.86 (.67)
T ≥ 80, P ≥ 85	.62	.88	.57	.59 (.31)	.87 (.69)
T ≥ 80, P ≥ 90	.57	.80	.60	.59 (.29)	.81 (.54)
T ≥ 80, P ≥ 93	.55	.80	.63	.61 (.32)	.81 (.56)
T ≥ 80, P ≥ 98	.37	.56	.77	.64 (.38)	.71 (.31)
T ≥ 85, P ≥ 80	.53	.84	.69	.66 (.41)	.86 (.66)
T ≥ 85, P ≥ 85	.52	.84	.71	.68 (.45)	.86 (.67)
T ≥ 85, P ≥ 90	.47	.76	.74	.68 (.45)	.81 (.55)
T ≥ 85, P ≥ 93	.45	.76	.77	.70 (.49)	.82 (.56)
T ≥ 85, P ≥ 98	.28	.52	.88	.76 (.60)	.72 (.33)
T ≥ 90, P ≥ 80	.48	.80	.74	.68 (.47)	.84 (.61)
T ≥ 90, P ≥ 85	.47	.80	.77	.71 (.51)	.84 (.63)
T ≥ 90, P ≥ 90	.42	.72	.80	.72 (.52)	.80 (.52)
T ≥ 90, P ≥ 93	.40	.72	.83	.75 (.57)	.81 (.53)
T ≥ 90, P ≥ 98	.25	.48	.91	.80 (.66)	.71 (.31)
		Differentiating ADHD/COM from ADHD/I			
T ≥ 80, P ≥ 80	.67	.88	.50	.59 (.26)	.83 (.63)
T ≥ 80, P ≥ 85	.67	.88	.50	.59 (.26)	.83 (.63)
T ≥ 80, P ≥ 90	.64	.80	.50	.57 (.21)	.75 (.45)
T ≥ 80, P ≥ 93	.60	.80	.57	.61 (.28)	.77 (.50)
T ≥ 80, P ≥ 98	.35	.56	.83	.74 (.52)	.69 (.33)
T ≥ 85, P ≥ 80	.55	.84	.70	.70 (.45)	.84 (.65)
T ≥ 85, P ≥ 85	.55	.84	.70	.70 (.45)	.84 (.65)
T ≥ 85, P ≥ 90	.51	.76	.70	.68 (.41)	.78 (.51)
T ≥ 85, P ≥ 93	.47	.76	.77	.73 (.51)	.79 (.54)
T ≥ 85, P ≥ 98	.27	.52	.93	.87 (.76)	.70 (.34)
T ≥ 90, P ≥ 80	.45	.80	.83	.80 (.63)	.83 (.63)
T ≥ 90, P ≥ 85	.45	.80	.83	.80 (.63)	.83 (.63)
T ≥ 90, P ≥ 90	.42	.72	.83	.78 (.60)	.78 (.52)
T ≥ 90, P ≥ 93	.40	.72	.87	.82 (.67)	.79 (.53)
T ≥ 90, P ≥ 98	.24	.48	.97	.92 (.86)	.69 (.32)

Note. From Power, Doherty, et al. (1998). Copyright 1998 by Plenum Publishing Corporation. Reprinted with permission from Springer Science + Business Media.

than the 80th percentile and parent ratings less than the 85th percentile had the most utility.

The Hyperactivity–Impulsivity subscale had limited utility in differentiating the ADHD/COM group from the control group. Alternatively, this subscale was useful in differentiating the ADHD/COM group from the ADHD/I group. The optimal approach to diagnosing ADHD/COM when ADHD/COM and ADHD/I were compared was a single-informant strategy using teacher ratings at or above the 93rd percentile on the Hyperactivity–Impulsivity subscale. The most useful approach to ruling out ADHD/COM when the two presentations were compared

TABLE 5.5. Optimal Cutoff Scores for Diagnosing and Ruling Out ADHD: Clinic-Based Study

Diagnosing ADHD/I	Inattention subscale (teacher) ≥ 90th percentile AND Inattention subscale (parent) ≥ 93rd percentile AND Hyperactivity–Impulsivity subscale (teacher) ≤ 80th percentile
Screening for ADHD/I	Inattention subscale (teacher) < 80th percentile AND Inattention subscale (parent) < 85th percentile Alternatively, Inattention subscale (parent) < 90th percentile
Diagnosing ADHD/COM	Inattention subscale (teacher) ≥ 90th percentile AND Inattention subscale (parent) ≥ 93rd percentile AND Hyperactivity–Impulsivity subscale (teacher) ≥ 93rd percentile
Ruling out ADHD/COM	Inattention subscale (teacher) < 80th percentile AND Inattention subscale (parent) < 85th percentile AND Hyperactivity–Impulsivity subscale (teacher) < 80th percentile Alternatively, Inattention subscale (parent) < 80th percentile AND Hyperactivity–Impulsivity subscale (parent) < 80th percentile

Note. The informant is indicated in parentheses.

also appeared to be a single-informant approach using teacher ratings below the 80th percentile on the Hyperactivity–Impulsivity subscale.

In clinical settings it is sometimes challenging to obtain teacher ratings of ADHD symptoms. In these cases, clinicians often must rely primarily on parent ratings. Fortunately, parent ratings were found to be useful in screening for or ruling out ADHD. When using parent ratings to screen for ADHD/I, the optimal approach was to use a cutoff point of the 90th percentile. When screening for ADHD/COM, the optimal cutoff points are ratings on both the Inattention and Hyperactivity–Impulsivity subscales less than the 80th percentile, as rated by parents.

Given that the Inattention subscale generally was more useful than the Hyperactivity–Impulsivity subscale in differentiating children with ADHD from those in the control group, a helpful strategy is to decide first whether a referred child has a disorder of inattention (either ADHD/I or ADHD/COM), using the Inattention subscale. The optimal cutoff scores reported in Table 5.5 should be helpful in making this determination. Next, if the clinician determines that the child has ADHD/I or ADHD/COM, the Hyperactivity–Impulsivity subscale can be very useful in identifying the most appropriate presentation, using the recommended cutoff scores delineated in Table 5.5.

It is important to note that 24% of children who actually had ADHD/COM and 43% of children who had ADHD/I were missed when the optimal cutoff scores on the Inattention subscale determined in this study were used. Moreover, in 36% of the cases, the Hyperactivity–Impulsivity subscale failed to sort out who had ADHD/COM versus ADHD/I when the optimal cutoff score on the teacher rating scale was used. Thus clinicians need to be cautious when using teacher and parent ratings of DSM symptoms to determine whether ADHD exists and what presentation is most descriptive of the child. Another reason for caution, as noted previously, is that the findings from the study reported in this chapter were derived using the ADHD Rating Scale–IV and not the current version of the scale.

At this point, a strategy that incorporates teacher and parent symptom ratings on the ADHD Rating Scale–5 along with informant ratings of symptom-related impairment and information derived from other measures (e.g., diagnostic interviews and behavioral observations, if feasible) is recommended in the diagnostic assessment of ADHD.

Given that there were so few children with ADHD/HI in this sample, it was not possible to investigate the ability of the Hyperactivity–Impulsivity subscale to differentiate children with ADHD/HI from controls. A useful guideline at this point is to consider the possibility of a diagnosis of ADHD/HI when (1) the inattentive or combined presentation of ADHD can be ruled out (i.e., teacher ratings on the Inattention subscale are less than the 80th percentile and parent ratings on this scale are less than the 85th percentile); and (2) teacher ratings of Hyperactivity–Impulsivity are greater than or equal to the 93rd percentile.

The results of this study are generalizable to clinic-based settings serving children in the age range from 6 to 14 years. The findings may be less applicable in other settings, including school-based programs and clinics serving preschool children or older adolescents. Use of the kappa correction statistics for PPP and NPP mitigates variations in predictability across settings that have differential base rates for symptoms and disorders (Chen et al., 1994; Frick et al., 1994). However, fundamental differences between settings in regard to referral agent (parent vs. teacher) and type of functional impairment may result in cross-situational inconsistencies in prediction that are not entirely corrected by kappa statistics. In using the ADHD Rating Scale–5 to make clinical decisions regarding children referred by teachers in a school setting, the guidelines described in the following sections should be more accurate and useful. Furthermore, clinicians need to be cautious about using the recommended cutoff scores in Table 5.5 with children who belong to racial/ethnic minority groups, especially children from African American backgrounds (see Chapter 3).

Finally, it should be noted that determinations about the diagnosis of ADHD require a consideration of symptom-related impairments and possible exclusionary conditions (American Psychiatric Association, 2013). With regard to the impairment criterion, based on the results of our research using the ADHD Rating Scale–5 (Power et al., 2015), an endorsement (i.e., rating of 2 = moderate impairment or 3 = severe impairment) of at least one parent-rated impairment and at least three teacher-rated impairments is generally recommended to support a possible diagnosis of ADHD.

Prediction in a School-Based Setting

Clinical Utility of the Inattention Subscale in a School Setting

Participants in the teacher-referred, school-based study included children in kindergarten through grade 8. Symptom utility estimates, including base rate, sensitivity, specificity, PPP, cPPP, NPP, and cNPP, for several possible cutoff scores (80th, 85th, 90th, 93rd, and 98th percentiles) on the Inattention subscale, as rated by teachers and parents, were computed. These are presented in Table 5.6. The strategy for determining optimal thresholds was to identify the cutoff score associated

TABLE 5.6. Symptom Utility Estimates Associated with Cutoff Scores on the Inattention Subscale: School-Based Study

Cutoff score	Base rate	Sensitivity	Specificity	PPP (cPPP)	NPP (cNPP)
		Differentiating ADHD/I from controls–Teacher ratings			
≥ 98	.06	.14	.97	.67 (.54)	.75 (.09)
≥ 93	.16	.34	.91	.59 (.43)	.78 (.22)
≥ 90	.21	.45	.88	.59 (.43)	.81 (.30)
≥ 85	.30	.59	.82	.55 (.38)	.84 (.41)
≥ 80	.42	.86	.75	.57 (.40)	.93 (.76)
		Differentiating ADHD/COM from controls–Teacher ratings			
≥ 98	.03	.04	.97	.33 (.13)	.77 (.01)
≥ 93	.15	.35	.91	.53 (.39)	.82 (.23)
≥ 90	.22	.57	.88	.59 (.47)	.87 (.44)
≥ 85	.31	.74	.82	.55 (.41)	.91 (.62)
≥ 80	.37	.78	.75	.49 (.33)	.92 (.65)
		Differentiating ADHD/I from controls–Parent ratings			
≥ 98	.11	.28	.95	.67 (.54)	.77 (.18)
≥ 93	.29	.48	.79	.47 (.26)	.80 (.28)
≥ 90	.36	.59	.72	.45 (.24)	.82 (.35)
≥ 85	.55	.76	.53	.38 (.14)	.85 (.46)
≥ 80	.67	.90	.41	.36 (.12)	.91 (.68)
		Differentiating ADHD/COM from controls–Parent ratings			
≥ 98	.11	.30	.95	.64 (.53)	.82 (.22)
≥ 93	.30	.61	.79	.47 (.31)	.87 (.44)
≥ 90	.38	.74	.72	.45 (.28)	.90 (.58)
≥ 85	.57	.91	.53	.37 (.18)	.95 (.80)
≥ 80	.66	.96	.41	.32 (.12)	.97 (.87)

with the highest level of accurate prediction (cPPP or cNPP) that resulted in a reasonable level of sensitivity or specificity. For purposes of this study, a cutoff score was considered clinically useful if cPPP or cNPP was greater than or equal to .65 and sensitivity or specificity was approximately .50 or greater.

Prediction Based on a Single Informant

The results indicated that single-informant ratings of Inattention were not useful in diagnosing ADHD/I or ADHD/COM. When the Inattention subscale was used to differentiate children with ADHD/I and ADHD/COM from those in the control group, cPPP statistics were well below an acceptable level at each of the cutoff scores examined, as rated by both teachers and parents, even though in some cases specificity values were high. For example, although teacher ratings below the 90th percentile were useful in detecting 88% of the children who had not met the criteria for ADHD/COM versus the control group (specificity), only 59% of children who scored at or above this cutoff score were diagnosed with ADHD/COM (PPP), resulting in a cPPP value of .47.

In contrast, parent and teacher ratings on the Inattention subscale, used separately, generally were highly useful in ruling out diagnoses. Teacher ratings below the 80th percentile were able to rule out ADHD/I in 93% of the cases (cNPP = .76), and 86% of the cases with a diagnosis of ADHD scored above this cutoff score (sensitivity). In addition, the specificity value associated with this cutoff was relatively high (.75). The same cutoff score was also able to rule out ADHD/COM in 92% of the cases (cNPP = .65) with a sensitivity of .78 and specificity of .75. Parent ratings on the Inattention subscale were also useful in ruling out ADHD/I and ADHD/COM, but they appeared somewhat less useful than teacher ratings. Parent ratings below the 80th percentile were able to rule out ADHD/I in 91% of the cases (cNPP = .68) with a sensitivity of .90, but the specificity associated with this cutoff score was only .41. Similarly, this cutoff score was able to rule out ADHD/COM in 97% of the cases (cNPP = .87) with a sensitivity of .96, but the specificity was .41.

Prediction Based on Multiple Informants

Given the results of logistic regression analyses demonstrating that the combination of teacher and parent ratings on the Inattention subscale was more effective than a single-informant approach in differentiating children with ADHD/I and ADHD/COM from those in the control group (see Chapter 4), symptom utility estimates for all possible combinations of teacher and parent ratings were computed. In general, the combination cutoff scores were better than the single-informant thresholds in predicting or ruling in ADHD/I and ADHD/COM. The combination cutoff scores that had the highest level of utility in predicting ADHD presentation are presented in Table 5.7. Combinations involving teacher ratings greater than or equal to the 93rd percentile were not included because these were associated with very low rates of sensitivity and cNPP. For the prediction of both ADHD/I and ADHD/COM, the optimal combination was a teacher rating at or above the 90th percentile and a parent rating at or above the 80th percentile. In predicting a diagnosis of ADHD/I, this combination of scores was associated with a cPPP of .65 and a specificity of .95, but sensitivity was only .41. For predicting a diagnosis of ADHD/COM, this combination yielded a cPPP value of .67, a specificity of .95, and a sensitivity of .52. Thus the optimal combination of cutoff values had a moderately high rate of prediction but failed to predict about 50% of the children who had ADHD/I or ADHD/COM. Combining teacher and parent ratings on the Inattention subscale was not as useful as a single-informant approach in screening for or ruling out ADHD.

Clinical Utility of the Hyperactivity–Impulsivity Subscale in a School Setting

Prediction Based on a Single Informant

Symptom utility estimates for several possible cutoff scores (80th, 85th, 90th, 93rd, and 98th percentiles) on the Hyperactivity–Impulsivity subscale of the ADHD

TABLE 5.7. Symptom Utility Estimates Associated with the Combination of Teacher (T) and Parent (P) Ratings on the Inattention Subscale: School-Based Study

Cutoff score	Base rate	Sensitivity	Specificity	PPP (cPPP)	NPP (cNPP)
		Differentiating ADHD/I from controls			
T ≥ 80, P ≥ 80	.32	.76	.84	.65 (.51)	.90 (.64)
T ≥ 80, P ≥ 85	.27	.66	.88	.68 (.56)	.87 (.53)
T ≥ 80, P ≥ 90	.20	.52	.92	.71 (.61)	.83 (.40)
T ≥ 80, P ≥ 93	.17	.45	.93	.72 (.62)	.82 (.33)
T ≥ 80, P ≥ 98	.09	.24	.97	.78 (.69)	.77 (.17)
T ≥ 85, P ≥ 80	.21	.70	.91	.68 (.56)	.83 (.39)
T ≥ 85, P ≥ 85	.18	.70	.92	.68 (.56)	.81 (.33)
T ≥ 85, P ≥ 90	.13	.61	.93	.64 (.51)	.78 (.20)
T ≥ 85, P ≥ 93	.12	.48	.95	.69 (.57)	.78 (.21)
T ≥ 85, P ≥ 98	.06	.22	.99	.83 (.77)	.76 (.12)
T ≥ 90, P ≥ 80	.15	.41	.95	.75 (.65)	.81 (.31)
T ≥ 90, P ≥ 85	.13	.34	.95	.71 (.61)	.79 (.24)
T ≥ 90, P ≥ 90	.10	.24	.95	.64 (.50)	.77 (.15)
T ≥ 90, P ≥ 93	.10	.24	.95	.64 (.50)	.77 (.15)
T ≥ 90, P ≥ 98	.05	.14	.99	.80 (.72)	.75 (.09)
		Differentiating ADHD/COM from controls			
T ≥ 80, P ≥ 80	.29	.74	.84	.59 (.46)	.91 (.63)
T ≥ 80, P ≥ 85	.25	.70	.88	.64 (.53)	.91 (.59)
T ≥ 80, P ≥ 90	.20	.61	.92	.70 (.61)	.89 (.51)
T ≥ 80, P ≥ 93	.16	.48	.93	.69 (.59)	.86 (.38)
T ≥ 80, P ≥ 98	.07	.22	.97	.71 (.63)	.80 (.16)
T ≥ 85, P ≥ 80	.23	.70	.91	.70 (.60)	.91 (.60)
T ≥ 85, P ≥ 85	.22	.70	.92	.73 (.64)	.91 (.61)
T ≥ 85, P ≥ 90	.18	.61	.93	.74 (.66)	.89 (.52)
T ≥ 85, P ≥ 93	.15	.48	.95	.73 (.65)	.86 (.39)
T ≥ 85, P ≥ 98	.06	.22	.99	.83 (.78)	.81 (.17)
T ≥ 90, P ≥ 80	.16	.52	.95	.75 (.67)	.87 (.43)
T ≥ 90, P ≥ 85	.16	.52	.95	.75 (.67)	.87 (.43)
T ≥ 90, P ≥ 90	.15	.48	.95	.73 (.65)	.86 (.39)
T ≥ 90, P ≥ 93	.13	.39	.95	.69 (.60)	.84 (.30)
T ≥ 90, P ≥ 98	.06	.22	.99	.83 (.78)	.81 (.17)

Note. From Power, Andrews, et al. (1998). Copyright 1998 by the American Psychological Association. Reprinted by permission.

Rating Scale–5, as rated by teachers and parents, were computed and are presented in Table 5.8. Teacher ratings of hyperactivity–impulsivity generally were not useful in predicting or ruling in diagnostic group membership. Parent ratings at or above the 98th percentile on the Hyperactivity–Impulsivity subscale were able to differentiate children with ADHD/COM from the control group at a moderate to high level (cPPP = .67 and specificity of .97), but only 26% of children with ADHD/COM scored above this cutoff score on the ADHD Rating Scale–IV (sensitivity). However, it should be noted that parent ratings at or above the 90th percentile were quite useful in predicting children with ADHD/COM as opposed

TABLE 5.8. Symptom Utility Estimates Associated with Cutoff Scores on the Hyperactivity–Impulsivity Subscale: School-Based Study

Cutoff score	Base rate	Sensitivity	Specificity	PPP (cPPP)	NPP (cNPP)
	Differentiating ADHD/COM from controls—Teacher ratings				
≥ 98	.04	.09	.97	.50 (.35)	.78 (.05)
≥ 93	.09	.22	.95	.56 (.42)	.80 (.14)
≥ 90	.12	.30	.93	.58 (.46)	.82 (.21)
≥ 85	.20	.48	.88	.55 (.41)	.85 (.35)
≥ 80	.28	.61	.82	.50 (.35)	.87 (.45)
	Differentiating ADHD/COM from ADHD/I—Teacher ratings				
≥ 98	.06	.09	.97	.67 (.40)	.57 (.03)
≥ 93	.17	.22	.86	.56 (.20)	.58 (.05)
≥ 90	.21	.30	.86	.64 (.35)	.61 (.12)
≥ 85	.33	.48	.79	.65 (.37)	.66 (.22)
≥ 80	.46	.61	.66	.58 (.25)	.68 (.27)
	Differentiating ADHD/COM from controls—Parent ratings				
≥ 98	.08	.26	.97	.75 (.67)	.81 (.20)
≥ 93	.21	.52	.88	.57 (.44)	.86 (.39)
≥ 90	.30	.65	.80	.50 (.35)	.88 (.50)
≥ 85	.39	.78	.72	.46 (.30)	.92 (.64)
≥ 80	.48	.87	.63	.42 (.24)	.94 (.75)
	Differentiating ADHD/COM from ADHD/I—Parent ratings				
≥ 98	.15	.26	.93	.75 (.55)	.61 (.13)
≥ 93	.29	.52	.90	.80 (.64)	.70 (.33)
≥ 90	.35	.65	.90	.83 (.70)	.76 (.47)
≥ 85	.50	.78	.72	.69 (.45)	.81 (.57)
≥ 80	.60	.87	.62	.65 (.36)	.86 (.68)

to ADHD/I; with the use of this cutoff score cPPP was .70, specificity was .90, and sensitivity was .65.

Parent ratings on the Hyperactivity–Impulsivity subscale were useful in ruling out diagnostic group membership, but teacher ratings were not. Parent ratings below the 80th percentile were able to rule out ADHD/COM in 94% of the cases (cNPP = .75) with a sensitivity of .87 and specificity of .63. Parent ratings below this cutoff score were also able to rule out the Combined presentation, when children with ADHD/I were compared with those with ADHD/COM, in 86% of the cases (cNPP = .68) with a sensitivity of .87 and specificity of .62.

Prediction Based on Multiple Informants

Given the results of logistic regression analyses demonstrating that the combination of teacher and parent ratings on the Hyperactivity–Impulsivity subscale was more effective than a single-informant approach in differentiating children with ADHD/COM from those in the control group, but not differentiating children with ADHD/COM from those with ADHD/I (see Chapter 4), symptom utility estimates for all possible combinations of teacher and parent ratings were computed. In general, the combination cutoff scores were better than the single-informant thresholds in predicting or ruling in subtype membership. The combination cutoff scores that had the highest level of utility in predicting subtype membership are presented in Table 5.9. Combinations involving teacher ratings greater than or equal to the 93rd percentile were not included because these were associated

TABLE 5.9. Symptom Utility Estimates Associated with the Combination of Teacher (T) and Parent (P) Ratings on the Hyperactivity–Impulsivity Subscale: School-Based Study

Cutoff score	Base rate	Sensitivity	Specificity	PPP (cPPP)	NPP (cNPP)
		Differentiating ADHD/COM from controls			
T ≥ 80, P ≥ 80	.16	.52	.95	.75 (.67)	.87 (.43)
T ≥ 80, P ≥ 85	.15	.52	.96	.80 (.74)	.87 (.44)
T ≥ 80, P ≥ 90	.12	.39	.96	.75 (.67)	.84 (.31)
T ≥ 80, P ≥ 93	.09	.30	.97	.78 (.71)	.82 (.23)
T ≥ 80, P ≥ 98	.03	.13	1.00	1.00 (1.00)	.79 (.10)
T ≥ 85, P ≥ 80	.13	.43	.96	.77 (.70)	.85 (.35)
T ≥ 85, P ≥ 85	.12	.43	.97	.83 (.78)	.85 (.36)
T ≥ 85, P ≥ 90	.09	.30	.97	.78 (.71)	.82 (.23)
T ≥ 85, P ≥ 93	.07	.22	.97	.71 (.63)	.80 (.16)
T ≥ 85, P ≥ 98	.02	.09	1.00	1.00 (1.00)	.78 (.07)
T ≥ 90, P ≥ 80	.08	.26	.97	.75 (.67)	.81 (.20)
T ≥ 90, P ≥ 85	.08	.26	.97	.75 (.67)	.81 (.20)
T ≥ 90, P ≥ 90	.06	.17	.97	.67 (.57)	.80 (.12)
T ≥ 90, P ≥ 93	.05	.13	.97	.60 (.48)	.79 (.08)
T ≥ 90, P ≥ 98	.02	.09	1.00	1.00 (1.00)	.78 (.07)
		Differentiating ADHD/COM from ADHD/I			
T ≥ 80, P ≥ 80	.27	.52	.93	.86 (.74)	.71 (.35)
T ≥ 80, P ≥ 85	.25	.52	.97	.92 (.86)	.72 (.36)
T ≥ 80, P ≥ 90	.19	.39	.97	.90 (.82)	.67 (.25)
T ≥ 80, P ≥ 93	.15	.30	.97	.88 (.78)	.64 (.18)
T ≥ 80, P ≥ 98	.08	.13	.97	.75 (.55)	.58 (.06)
T ≥ 85, P ≥ 80	.21	.43	.97	.91 (.84)	.68 (.28)
T ≥ 85, P ≥ 85	.19	.43	1.00	1.00 (1.00)	.69(.30)
T ≥ 85, P ≥ 90	.13	.30	1.00	1.00 (1.00)	.64 (.20)
T ≥ 85, P ≥ 93	.10	.22	1.00	1.00 (1.00)	.62 (.13)
T ≥ 85, P ≥ 98	.04	.09	1.00	1.00 (1.00)	.58 (.05)
T ≥ 90, P ≥ 80	.12	.26	1.00	1.00 (1.00)	.63 (.16)
T ≥ 90, P ≥ 85	.12	.26	1.00	1.00 (1.00)	.63 (.16)
T ≥ 90, P ≥ 90	.08	.17	1.00	1.00 (1.00)	.60 (.11)
T ≥ 90, P ≥ 93	.06	.13	1.00	1.00 (1.00)	.59 (.08)
T ≥ 90, P ≥ 98	.04	.09	1.00	1.00 (1.00)	.58 (.05)

Note. From Power, Andrews, et al. (1998). Copyright 1998 by the American Psychological Association. Reprinted by permission.

with very low rates of sensitivity and cNPP. For the prediction of ADHD/COM, the optimal combination was a teacher rating at or above the 80th percentile and a parent rating at or above the 85th percentile. In predicting children with ADHD/COM as compared with the control group, this combination of scores was associated with a cPPP of .74, a specificity of .96, and a sensitivity of .52. For predicting children with ADHD/COM as compared with those with ADHD/I, this combination yielded a cPPP value of .86, a specificity of .97, and a sensitivity of .52. Thus the optimal combination of cutoff values had a high rate of prediction but failed to predict about 50% of the children who had ADHD/COM. Combining teacher and parent ratings on the Hyperactivity–Impulsivity subscale was not as useful as a single-informant approach in ruling out diagnoses of ADHD.

Conclusions: Prediction in a School Setting

Optimal cutoff scores for diagnosing and ruling out ADHD in our teacher-referred, school-based sample are summarized in Table 5.10. The results pointed to the conclusion that in a school-based sample of children referred by teachers, a single-informant approach for each ADHD dimension is best for ruling out ADHD, whereas an approach that combines parent and teacher ratings for each ADHD dimension is more useful in diagnosing this disorder. The results further suggested that teacher and parent reports of ADHD symptoms, as assessed by the ADHD Rating Scale–5, may be more useful in screening for ADHD than diagnosing this disorder, unless additional measures are used for diagnosis.

The Inattention subscale, rated by either teachers or parents, was quite successful in ruling out children with ADHD/I and ADHD/COM, although teacher reports appeared somewhat more accurate and useful than parent reports. Ratings by teachers below the 80th percentile on the Inattention subscale were optimal in ruling out ADHD. The combined-informant approach was more successful in predicting the presence of ADHD than the single-informant approach. For example, teacher ratings on the Inattention subscale at or above the 90th percentile were accurate in predicting ADHD/COM 59% of the time (cPPP = .47). However, when

TABLE 5.10. Optimal Cutoff Scores for Diagnosing and Ruling Out ADHD in the Teacher-Referred, School-Based Sample: School-Based Study

Diagnosing ADHD/I	Inattention subscale (teacher) ≥ 90th percentile AND Inattention subscale (parent) ≥ 80th percentile AND Hyperactivity–Impulsivity subscale (parent) ≤ 80th percentile
Ruling out ADHD/I	Inattention subscale (teacher) < 80th percentile
Diagnosing ADHD/COM	Inattention subscale (teacher) ≥ 90th percentile AND Inattention subscale (parent) ≥ 80th percentile AND Hyperactivity–Impulsivity subscale (teacher) ≥ 80th percentile AND Hyperactivity–Impulsivity subscale (parent) ≥ 85th percentile
Ruling out ADHD/COM	Inattention subscale (teacher) < 80th percentile AND Hyperactivity–Impulsivity subscale (parent) < 80th percentile

Note. The informant is indicated in parentheses.

teacher ratings at or above the 90th percentile were combined with parent ratings at or above the 80th percentile, the prediction rate increased to 75% (cPPP = .65 to .67). Although prediction was improved with the combined-informant approach resulting in a specificity value of .95, cPPP was only moderately high and sensitivity was relatively low.

The Hyperactivity–Impulsivity subscale rated by parents, but not by teachers, was useful in ruling out a diagnosis of ADHD/COM. Parent ratings at or below the 80th percentile resulted in a moderate to high level of predictive power (cNPP of .68 to .75), a high level of sensitivity (.87), and a reasonable level of specificity (.62 to .63). For predicting or ruling in ADHD/COM, the combined informant approach using the Hyperactivity–Impulsivity subscale demonstrated superiority over a single-informant approach. For example, teacher ratings on the Hyperactivity–Impulsivity subscale at or above the 80th percentile were successful in differentiating between children in the ADHD/COM group and children in the control group 50% of the time (cPPP = .35). However, when teacher ratings at or above the 80th percentile were combined with parent ratings at or above the 85th percentile, the prediction rate increased to 80% (cPPP = .74). This combination was associated with a high specificity value (.96), but a relatively low sensitivity rate (.52).

The ADHD Rating Scale–5 appears to be most useful in a school setting as a screening measure to be included in a multi-gate assessment process. Teacher ratings of Inattention were more useful than parent ratings in ruling out a disorder involving inattention (ADHD/I and ADHD/COM); parent ratings of hyperactivity–impulsivity were more useful than teacher ratings in ruling out ADHD/COM. The results of this study generally do not support the practice of using teacher and parent ratings alone or in combination in making diagnostic decisions about the presence of ADHD. Even though using a combination of teacher and parent reports of ADHD symptoms yielded a more accurate prediction of the presence of ADHD than a single-informant approach, predictive power and sensitivity generally were not high when the combined method was used, particularly when the Inattention subscale was used to predict ADHD/I and ADHD/COM. A more sensible approach is to use teacher and parent ratings in conjunction with other methods, such as informant ratings of symptom-related impairment, diagnostic interviews, and direct observation procedures, in making diagnostic decisions about ADHD. Given that there were no students in this sample who had ADHD/HI, it was not possible to evaluate the ability of the ADHD Rating Scale–5 to predict this presentation. A useful guideline at this point is to consider the possibility of a diagnosis of ADHD/HI when an Inattentive presentation of ADHD can be ruled out (i.e., teacher ratings on the Inattention subscale are less than the 80th percentile), and ratings scales indicate that a hyperactive–impulsive presentation of ADHD is likely (i.e., teacher ratings on the Hyperactivity–Impulsivity subscale are greater than or equal to the 80th percentile and parent ratings on this subscale are greater than or equal to the 85th percentile).

The results of this study are generalizable to samples of children referred to school-based pre-referral intervention teams for attention, learning, and behavior problems. The use of kappa correction statistics for PPP and NPP mitigates variations in predictability across settings that have different base rates for symptoms and disorders (Chen et al., 1994; Frick et al., 1994). Nonetheless, it is possible that differences between settings (e.g., psychiatric clinic vs. school-based team) in regard to referral agent and primary areas of functional impairment may result in cross-situational differences that cannot be entirely corrected statistically. Additional research is needed to identify the optimal approach to using teacher and parent report data among samples of referred children that differ by setting, referral source, and primary areas of functional impairment. As indicated earlier in this chapter, clinicians must be careful about using recommended cutoff scores in making clinical decisions about children belonging to ethnic minority groups. Also, the findings reported in this chapter need to be applied with caution in interpreting the ADHD Rating Scale–5 because they were derived from research conducted using the previous version of this measure.

As indicated previously, determinations about the diagnosis of ADHD require a consideration of symptom-related impairments. Based on our research using the ADHD Rating Scale–5 (Power et al., 2015), an endorsement (i.e., rating of 2 = moderate impairment or 3 = severe impairment) of at least one parent-rated impairment and at least three teacher-rated impairments is generally recommended to support a possible diagnosis of ADHD.

Case Examples

Darnell

Darnell is an 8-year-old boy who was referred to a hospital-based clinic by his parents because of their concerns about his inattention and behavior problems. Darnell is an African American student who lives in a poor, urban environment. Teacher ratings on the ADHD Rating Scale–5 indicated that he was at the 93rd percentile on the Inattention subscale and at the 90th percentile on the Hyperactivity–Impulsivity subscale. In addition, the teacher noted moderate or severe symptom-related impairments in the areas of teacher relationships, peer relationships, and homework performance. His mother rated him on this measure at the 93rd percentile for Inattention and at the 85th percentile for Hyperactivity–Impulsivity. Furthermore, the mother rated Darnell as having moderate or severe symptom-related impairments in the areas of peer relationships and homework performance. Given that ratings from teachers and parents on the Inattention subscale were above the optimal cutoff scores for diagnosing or ruling in ADHD/COM and ADHD/I in a parent-referred clinic setting (see Table 5.5), and given the presence of three teacher-rated and two parent-rated impairments, it is likely that Darnell meets the criteria for ADHD. Alternatively, given that research has shown that teacher ratings for black students generally are somewhat higher than for white students (DuPaul, Reid, Anastopoulos, & Power, 2014), clinicians should interpret normative data and recommended cutoff scores cautiously. Furthermore, because teacher ratings on the Hyperactivity–Impulsivity subscale were below the optimal cutoff score for predicting ADHD/COM (93rd percentile), it is unclear from rating scale data whether a diagnosis of ADHD/COM or ADHD/I is more appropriate. The clinician should interview the parent and review school information carefully to confirm that ADHD symptoms are contributing to functional problems at home and in school, and determine whether there is a sufficient level of hyperactivity–impulsivity to warrant a diagnosis of ADHD/COM versus ADHD/I.

Jennifer

Jennifer is an 11-year-old white girl living in a middle-class suburban neighborhood who was referred by her teacher to the school's pre-referral intervention team because of concerns related to attention, learning, and behavior problems. Teacher ratings on the ADHD Rating Scale–5 were at the 93rd percentile on the Inattention subscale and at the 50th percentile on the Hyperactivity–Impulsivity subscale. In addition, teachers reported symptom-related impairments in homework performance, academic performance, and self-esteem. Parent ratings were at the 90th percentile on the Inattention subscale and at the 75th percentile on the Hyperactivity–Impulsivity subscale. The parents reported symptom-related impairments in homework performance. Teacher and parent ratings on the Inattention subscale and the impairment scale strongly suggested the presence of ADHD (see Table 5.10). Because parent and teacher ratings on the Hyperactivity–Impulsivity subscale were relatively low and within the range where ADHD/COM could be ruled out, the data strongly suggest the presence of ADHD/I. The clinician should review assessment findings, and perhaps confer again with the parents and teachers, to confirm that symptoms of ADHD were elevated and contributing to impairments.

Robert

Robert is a 6-year-old white boy from a working-class neighborhood who was referred to a community-based clinic by his parents because of their concern about his learning and behavior problems. Teacher ratings on the ADHD Rating Scale–5 indicated that he was at the 93rd percentile on the Inattention subscale and at the 85th percentile on the Hyperactivity–Impulsivity subscale. In addition, the teacher noted symptom-related impairments in peer relationships and academic performance. Parent ratings on this measure placed Robert at the 85th percentile for Inattention and Hyperactivity–Impulsivity, and symptom-related impairments in academic performance. Teacher ratings of Inattention were above the optimal cutoff score for diagnosing ADHD, but parent ratings were not (see Table 5.5). Teacher and parent ratings on the Hyperactivity–Impulsivity subscale were not below the thresholds for ruling out ADHD/COM. Furthermore, parent and teacher reports both noted the presence of symptom-related impairments. In this case, the diagnosis is unclear, although Robert is clearly struggling with academic performance, which appears to be related in part to attention problems. It is recommended that the clinician confer again with the parents and teachers and review school information to sort out diagnostic issues. While diagnostic information is being sorted out, it is recommended that the clinician consult with the parents and teachers to develop a plan to address the child's academic and peer relationship concerns.

Maria

Maria, a 7-year-old Latina girl who lives in a rural setting, was referred by her teacher to the school's pre-referral intervention team because of concern about her attention and learning problems. Teacher ratings on the ADHD Rating Scale–5 were at the 75th percentile for Inattention and at the 75th percentile for Hyperactivity–Impulsivity. The teacher noted symptom-related impairments in academic and homework performance. Parent ratings on the Inattention subscale were at the 50th percentile and at the 75th percentile for Hyperactivity–Impulsivity. The parents also noted symptom-related impairments in academic and homework performance. Given that teacher and parent ratings on both the Inattention and Hyperactivity–Impulsivity subscales were below the cutoff scores for ruling out ADHD in a teacher-referred school sample (see Table 5.10), it is not likely that Maria meets the criteria for this disorder. Alternatively, both parent and teacher ratings of symptom-related impairments suggest that problems with attention and/or behavioral control may be contributing to academic difficulties. Before ruling out ADHD conclusively, the clinician should review the historical data presented by the family, conduct observations in the classroom if feasible, and carefully review school records. Regardless of diagnostic status, the clinician should consult with the parents and teachers to develop a plan to address the student's academic and homework problems.

CHAPTER 6

Interpretation and Use of the Scales for Evaluating Treatment Outcome

Many different types of evidence-based treatments have been identified for use with children and adolescents with ADHD. Included among these are various forms of pharmacotherapy, parenting and family-based interventions, school-based treatments, and summer treatment programming (Barkley, 2015; DuPaul & Stoner, 2014). Although many of these treatments are commonly used alone in clinical practice, research over the past several years has shown that greater clinical efficacy is achieved when such treatments are used in combination. Less clear from the research literature is any guidance for determining which treatment combinations work best for which individuals, for which target behaviors, and under which conditions. Thus it is not the case that treatments can merely be selected from a list of evidence-based interventions and then implemented in cookbook fashion. Instead, health care professionals must use some degree of clinical judgment in making such treatment determinations.

The necessity for using clinical judgment introduces an element of uncertainty into the process of implementing planned treatments. Even when using those treatments for which there is strong empirical support, there is no guarantee that therapeutic improvements will be achieved. Therefore, once intervention plans are set in motion, there remains an equally important but often overlooked clinical task to address—namely, determining whether treatment worked. Many different factors can influence one's conclusion as to whether an individual with ADHD has benefited from treatment. Because a thorough discussion of this matter is beyond the scope of this chapter, readers are encouraged to consider other sources (e.g., Anastopoulos & Shelton, 2011).

For the purposes of this manual, we focus our discussion on two important components of the process of assessing treatment outcome—namely, determining which behaviors should be targeted for treatment and which criterion should be used for assessing the impact of treatment.

Assessing the Clinical Significance of Treatment Outcome

In everyday clinical practice, the goal of treatment is primarily focused on ameliorating primary ADHD symptoms. Implicit in this approach is the idea that as primary ADHD symptoms are brought under better control, concomitant improvements in school performance, peer relations, and other domains of daily functioning will follow. Although intuitively appealing, support for this assumption has been less than compelling. Recently reported findings have shown an apparent disconnect between changes in ADHD symptoms and changes in daily functioning (Karpenko, Owens, Evangelista, & Dodds, 2009; Owens, Johannes, & Karpenko, 2009). More specifically, up to 40% of a group of children with ADHD showed reliable reductions in their primary ADHD symptoms in the absence of concurrent improvements in daily functioning. Moreover, 16% of the individuals in that same study showed improvements in functioning in the absence of any improvements in ADHD symptoms.

The take-home message from such findings is that clinicians and researchers who are interested in assessing treatment outcome should not focus exclusively on ADHD symptom reduction, as it may have limited bearing on addressing the kinds of functional impairments that accompany ADHD. Instead, to ensure that improved functioning has occurred, measures tapping into these functional outcomes must routinely be included in the process of assessing treatment response. As noted throughout this manual, the ADHD Rating Scale–5 is well suited to this purpose, as it allows for simultaneous assessment of changes in both ADHD symptoms and symptom-related functioning.

Ideally, treatment brings about clinically meaningful reductions in ADHD symptom levels that are accompanied by clinically meaningful improvements in the child's daily functioning. But how does one determine what is clinically meaningful? At its most fundamental level, clinically meaningful change can be defined in terms of whether a child's ADHD symptoms and daily functioning after treatment are similar to that of children of the same age and gender. For many children with ADHD, however, improvement to a level commensurate with peers may not always be realistic. Nonetheless, it remains important to interpret improvement in relation to a developmentally typical range of functioning.

So how does one determine the degree to which a child's behavior and functioning have been normalized? In clinical practice an especially common way to address these questions is simply to ask parents and teachers whether a particular treatment led to improvements both in the child's ADHD symptom presentation and in the child's home/school functioning. If the answer is "yes" to both questions, then the treatment worked; if "no," it did not. Obviously, this approach is highly subjective and, therefore, prone to numerous inaccuracies that can lead to faulty conclusions about treatment efficacy. A more objective way to address these same normative questions involves the use of parent- and teacher-completed behavior rating scales, or perhaps even psychological test procedures administered to the child directly or direct measures of child school performance, prior to and following treatment. Although quantifying change in this way certainly increases objectivity, there remains much room for subjective clinical judgment to enter into the decision-making process. To illustrate this point, should any change from pretreatment to posttreatment be considered evidence of clinically significant improvement? If not, of what magnitude should the change be before one can arrive at a conclusion that treatment was successful and produced a clinically meaningful outcome?

Fortunately, numerous statistical methods have been developed to assist clinicians and researchers in answering these questions. Of particular relevance for the purposes of this discussion is the Reliable Change Index (RCI) procedure for assessing clinical significance that was developed by Jacobsen and Truax (1991). According to this approach, the RCI is equal to the difference between a child's pretreatment score and posttreatment score, divided by the standard error of difference between the two test scores. When the RCI value exceeds 1.96, it is unlikely that the change from pretreatment to posttreatment is due to chance ($p < .05$). Thus the RCI serves as a measure of the degree to which improvement in functioning is likely due to the effects of treatment rather than to imprecise measurement.

$$\text{RCI} = \frac{\text{Posttreatment score} - \text{Pretreatment score}}{\text{Standard error of difference}}$$

The manner in which the ADHD Rating Scale–5 symptoms are scored and standardized is well suited to analysis using the RCI approach. To assist clinicians in making such determinations, we have calculated standard errors of difference for the Inattention, Hyperactivity–Impulsivity, and total scores according to age and gender groupings. The standard errors of difference for the School Version of ADHD Rating Scale–5 are presented in Table 6.1; those for the Home Version appear in Table 6.2. To calculate an RCI score for a specific child, one should first subtract the pretreatment rating scale score from the posttreatment score. The resulting difference score should then be divided by the corresponding standard error of difference, as displayed in Tables 6.1 and 6.2. For example, if one were attempting to calculate an RCI for teacher ratings of an 11-year-old boy on the Inattention subscale, the standard error of difference that would be used in the denominator would be 4.21 (see Table 6.1).

TABLE 6.1. Standard Errors of Difference for ADHD Rating Scale–5, School Version, Scores

Age (years)	Boys			Girls		
	IA	HI	Total	IA	HI	Total
5–7	3.34	3.14	5.02	2.94	2.73	4.60
8–10	3.48	3.23	5.45	2.77	2.11	3.90
11–13	4.21	4.00	5.29	3.75	2.88	4.23
14–17	3.77	3.70	4.81	2.71	2.15	3.12

Note. IA, Inattention; HI, Hyperactivity–Impulsivity.

TABLE 6.2. Standard Errors of Difference for ADHD Rating Scale-5, Home Version, Scores

	Boys			Girls		
Age (years)	IA	HI	Total	IA	HI	Total
5–7	3.66	3.12	5.26	3.30	2.90	4.80
8–10	3.42	3.25	5.20	3.31	2.47	4.41
11–13	4.75	4.18	8.10	4.07	3.55	6.83
14–17	4.59	3.11	7.20	4.53	3.18	7.24

Note. IA, Inattention; HI, Hyperactivity–Impulsivity.

The manner in which the ADHD Rating Scale–5 impairment ratings are scored and standardized is different than that for the symptom ratings, thereby necessitating an approach to assessing treatment outcome other than the RCI. In brief review (see Chapter 3), impairment is recorded as present for any of the six ADHD Rating Scale–5 impairment domains if an informant rates the item as a moderate or severe problem for either the Inattention or Hyperactivity–Impulsivity symptom clusters. The total number of impairments for any particular child can therefore range from 0 to 6. The frequency and cumulative percentages of impairments are displayed separately for parents and teachers in Table 3.9. As can be seen from this table, most children (87.6%) received 0 to 1 impairment ratings from parents; a similar percentage of children (87.4%) received 0 to 3 impairment ratings from teachers. On the basis of these and related findings (see Chapter 3), we have defined clinically significant impairment in terms of children having one or more parent-rated impairments and/or three or more teacher-rated impairments.

As mentioned earlier in this chapter, clinically meaningful change can be viewed in terms of whether a child's ADHD symptoms and daily functioning after treatment are within normal limits. In keeping with this conceptualization, the goal of treatment, therefore, is for a child to receive 0 parent-rated impairment ratings and no more than 2 teacher-rated impairment ratings following receipt of treatment services. Although up to 2 teacher-rated impairment ratings is not considered *statistically* significant based on the ADHD Rating Scale–5 normative table (see Table 3.9), the presence of any teacher rating suggesting moderate to severe impairment in any one domain should be taken seriously. In such situations, practitioners should use clinical judgment to determine the need for further evaluation and treatment.

Case Example

Brittany is a 10-year-old fifth-grade girl who was diagnosed with ADHD, Combined presentation. Like many other children with ADHD, Brittany's ADHD was accompanied by a comorbid diagnosis—namely, a specific learning disorder related to reading. To address this co-occurring learning condition, Brittany was receiving special education services in school, which had brought about improvements in her reading skills. Concerns remained, however, about the impact that her untreated ADHD was having on her behavior and daily functioning. Although she certainly exhibited ADHD symptoms and ADHD-related problems both at home and at school, most of her difficulties occurred in a classroom setting. For this reason, Brittany's parents agreed with her pediatrician's recommendation that she undergo a trial of stimulant medication therapy. Throughout the course of this 4-week trial Brittany was taking a medium dose of a commonly used long-acting stimulant medication, which she seemed to tolerate very well.

On two occasions—1 week prior to starting the medication trial and 1 week after completing it—Brittany's mother and teacher completed ADHD Rating Scale–5 ratings. For the purposes of this case discussion, only the teacher ADHD Rating Scale–5 ratings will be considered. Prior to starting medication, Brittany received the following ADHD symptom ratings from her teacher: an Inattention score of 24 and a Hyperactivity–Impulsivity score of 14, both of which were in the clinically significant range for her age and gender (see Symptom Scoring Sheet for Girls in the Appendix). Her teacher also indicated that Brittany was displaying moderate to severe impairment in four of the six ADHD Rating Scale–5 impairment domains, including Academics, Homework, Peer Relations, and Self-Esteem.

ADHD Rating Scale–5 ratings completed by the teacher in the week following the medication trial revealed improvements in some, but not all, areas. There was a marked reduction in Brittany's hyperactive–impulsive symptoms, which dropped from 14 to 8. To determine whether the magnitude of this change was clinically significant, an RCI score was calculated by dividing the difference between her pretreatment and posttreatment scores (14 – 8 = 6) by the corresponding standard error of difference (2.11) as reported in Table 6.1. This resulted in an RCI value of 2.84, which is above the recommended cutoff point of 1.96, thereby allowing for a determination that this improvement in Brittany's display of hyperactive–impulsive symptoms was in fact clinically significant. Although there was also improvement in Brittany's inattention symptoms, it was less clear at face value whether this change was clinically significant. Her inattention score decreased from 24 at pretreatment to 19 at posttreatment. This difference of 5, divided by the corresponding standard error of difference (2.77) listed in Table 6.1, yielded an RCI of 1.80. Thus it could not be concluded with any confidence that this change in her Inattention score was due to the effects of the medication rather than chance variation. Further complicating matters was that the teacher continued to rate Brittany as showing moderate to severe impairment in the same four areas of functioning—Academics, Homework, Peer Relations, and Self-Esteem—as had been the case prior to starting treatment.

Interpretation of these findings suggested that, while there was some evidence of clinically significant improvement from taking stimulant medication, Brittany's response to this treatment was insufficient. More specifically, in contrast with the clinically significant improvement in her hyperactive–impulsive symptoms, the change in her inattention symptoms could not be considered clinically significant. Moreover, neither of these reductions in ADHD symptoms was associated with a reduction in the number of functional impairments reported by her teacher. For there to be additional improvements in her levels of inattention and with respect to her four areas of impairment, her treatment plan needed to change. Initial consideration was given to increasing the dosage of her current stimulant medication, or perhaps even changing to another type of stimulant medication. Brittany and her parents decided not to change the medication regimen, given that it seemed to be somewhat beneficial, and opted to incorporate a comprehensive school-based intervention, which included use of a daily report card system and other evidence-based classroom strategies (DuPaul & Stoner, 2014), in combination with ongoing stimulant medication therapy.

Consistent with the format of the initial stimulant medication trial, teacher ADHD Rating Scale–5 ratings were once again obtained 1 month after instituting the school-based intervention. At this time Brittany's Inattention and Hyperactive–Impulsive scores were 12 and 6, respectively. Relative to her ADHD Rating Scale–5 symptom scores obtained at the end of the medication trial, these new results represented a change of 7 in Brittany's Inattention score and a change of 2 in her Hyperactive–Impulsive score. This difference of 7 in her display of inattention symptoms, divided by the corresponding standard error of difference (2.77) listed in Table 6.1, resulted in an RCI calculation of 2.53, suggesting that the addition of a school-based intervention to her treatment plan had brought about clinically meaningful change. In contrast, the decrease in her Hyperactive–Impulsive score, from 8 to 6, was not clinically significant based on a consideration of an RCI value of .95 that was calculated by dividing this difference (2) by the corresponding standard error of difference (2.11). The absence of clinically significant improvement in her hyperactive–impulsive symptoms was not a concern because her ongoing use of stimulant medication had reduced these symptoms to a level that was within normal limits for her age and gender (see ADHD Rating Scale–5, School Version: Symptom Scoring Sheet for Girls in the Appendix). Further examination of the ADHD Rating Scale–5 findings revealed that Brittany was now showing moderate to severe impairment in only one of the four areas of functioning (Peer Relations) that previously had been unresponsive to stimulant medication treatment alone. That there was no longer teacher-reported impairment in her Academics, Homework, and Self-Esteem very likely resulted from the addition of the comprehensive school-based intervention to her ongoing stimulant medication regimen. Moreover, this total number of teacher-reported impairments was not considered to be clinically significant, based on a consideration of the normative information listed for cumulative impairments in Table 3.9. That said, the fact that her teacher was still reporting that Brittany was having moderate to severe difficulties in her Peer Relations speaks to the need for further evaluation, and possibly to the need for initiating evidence-based treatment services that specifically target this area of concern.

APPENDIX

Rating Scales and Scoring Sheets

Attention and Behavior Rating Form, Home Version: Child (English)

Child's name: ______________________ Sex: M F Age: _______ Grade: ______________

Completed by: Mother ____ Father ____ Guardian ____ Grandparent ____

Please select the answer that *best describes your child's behavior over the past 6 months.*

How often does your child display this behavior?	Never or Rarely	Sometimes	Often	Very Often
Fails to give close attention to details or makes careless mistakes in schoolwork or during other activities	0	1	2	3
Has difficulty sustaining attention in tasks or play activities	0	1	2	3
Does not seem to listen when spoken to directly	0	1	2	3
Does not follow through on instructions and fails to finish schoolwork or chores	0	1	2	3
Has difficulty organizing tasks and activities	0	1	2	3
Avoids, dislikes, or is reluctant to engage in tasks that require sustained mental effort (e.g., schoolwork or homework)	0	1	2	3
Loses things necessary for tasks or activities (e.g., school materials, pencils, books, eyeglasses)	0	1	2	3
Easily distracted	0	1	2	3
Forgetful in daily activities (e.g., doing chores)	0	1	2	3

How much do the nine behaviors in the previous question cause problems for your child:	No Problem	Minor Problem	Moderate Problem	Severe Problem
Getting along with family members	0	1	2	3
Getting along with other children	0	1	2	3
Completing or returning homework	0	1	2	3
Performing academically in school	0	1	2	3
Controlling behavior in school	0	1	2	3
Feeling good about himself/herself	0	1	2	3

(continued)

How often does your child display this behavior?	Never or Rarely	Sometimes	Often	Very Often
Fidgets with or taps hands or feet or squirms in seat	0	1	2	3
Leaves seat in situations when remaining seated is expected	0	1	2	3
Runs about or climbs in situations where it is inappropriate	0	1	2	3
Unable to play or engage in leisure activities quietly	0	1	2	3
"On the go," acts as if "driven by a motor"	0	1	2	3
Talks excessively	0	1	2	3
Blurts out an answer before a question has been completed	0	1	2	3
Has difficulty waiting his or her turn (e.g., while waiting in line).	0	1	2	3
Interrupts or intrudes on others	0	1	2	3

How much do the nine behaviors in the previous question cause problems for your child:	No Problem	Minor Problem	Moderate Problem	Severe Problem
Getting along with family members	0	1	2	3
Getting along with other children	0	1	2	3
Completing or returning homework	0	1	2	3
Performing academically in school	0	1	2	3
Controlling behavior in school	0	1	2	3
Feeling good about him-/herself	0	1	2	3

Attention and Behavior Rating Form, Home Version: Adolescent (English)

Child's name: ______________________ Sex: M F Age: ________ Grade: ________________

Completed by: Mother ____ Father ____ Guardian ____ Grandparent ____

Please select the answer that *best describes your teenager's behavior over the past 6 months.*

How often does your child display this behavior?	Never or Rarely	Sometimes	Often	Very Often
Fails to give close attention to details or makes careless mistakes in schoolwork, at work, or during other activities	0	1	2	3
Has difficulty sustaining attention in tasks or play activities (e.g., has difficulty remaining focused during conversations or lengthy reading)	0	1	2	3
Does not seem to listen when spoken to directly	0	1	2	3
Does not follow through on instructions and fails to finish schoolwork, chores, or duties in the workplace	0	1	2	3
Has difficulty organizing tasks and activities	0	1	2	3
Avoids, dislikes, or is reluctant to engage in tasks that require sustained mental effort (e.g., schoolwork or homework; preparing reports)	0	1	2	3
Loses things necessary for tasks or activities (e.g., school materials, pencils, books, tools, wallets, keys, paperwork, eyeglasses, mobile telephones)	0	1	2	3
Easily distracted	0	1	2	3
Forgetful in daily activities (e.g., doing chores, running errands, returning calls, keeping appointments)	0	1	2	3

How much do the nine behaviors in the previous question cause problems for your teenager:	No Problem	Minor Problem	Moderate Problem	Severe Problem
Getting along with family members	0	1	2	3
Getting along with other teenagers	0	1	2	3
Completing or returning homework	0	1	2	3
Performing academically in school	0	1	2	3
Controlling behavior in school	0	1	2	3
Feeling good about himself/herself	0	1	2	3

(continued)

How often does your teenager display this behavior?	Never or Rarely	Sometimes	Often	Very Often
Fidgets with or taps hands or feet or squirms in seat	0	1	2	3
Leaves seat in situations when remaining seated is expected	0	1	2	3
Runs about or climbs in situations where it is inappropriate or feels restless	0	1	2	3
Unable to play or engage in leisure activities quietly (e.g., is unable to be or is uncomfortable being still for an extended period of time)	0	1	2	3
"On the go," acts as if "driven by a motor"	0	1	2	3
Talks excessively	0	1	2	3
Blurts out an answer before a question has been completed	0	1	2	3
Has difficulty waiting his or her turn (e.g., while waiting in line).	0	1	2	3
Interrupts or intrudes on others (e.g., butts into conversations, games, or activities; may intrude into or take over what others are doing)	0	1	2	3

How much do the nine behaviors in the previous question cause problems for your teenager:	No Problem	Minor Problem	Moderate Problem	Severe Problem
Getting along with family members	0	1	2	3
Getting along with other teenagers	0	1	2	3
Completing or returning homework	0	1	2	3
Performing academically in school	0	1	2	3
Controlling behavior in school	0	1	2	3
Feeling good about himself/herself	0	1	2	3

Attention and Behavior Rating Form, Home Version: Child (Spanish)

Edad del niño/niña:______________________ Sexo: M F Grado: _____ País de origen: ____________

Completado por: Madre ____ Padre ____ Abuela/o ____ Otro parentesco ____

Seleccione la respuesta *que describe mejor el comportamiento de su hijo/a en los últimos 6 meses.*

¿Con qué frecuencia su hijo/a tiene este comportamiento?	Nunca o rara vez	En ocasiones	A menudo	Con mucha frecuencia
Falla en prestar la debida atención a detalles o por descuido se cometen errores en las tareas escolares, o durante otras actividades	0	1	2	3
Tiene dificultades para mantener la atención en tareas o actividades recreativas	0	1	2	3
Parece no escuchar cuando se le habla directamente	0	1	2	3
No sigue las instrucciones y no termina las tareas escolares o los quehaceres	0	1	2	3
Tiene dificultad para organizar tareas y actividades	0	1	2	3
Evita, le disgusta o se muestra poco entusiasta en iniciar tareas que requieren un esfuerzo mental sostenido (p. ej., tareas escolares o quehaceres domésticos)	0	1	2	3
Pierde cosas necesarias para tareas o actividades (p. ej., materiales escolares, lápices, libros, gafas)	0	1	2	3
Se distrae con facilidad por estímulos externos	0	1	2	3
Olvida las actividades cotidianas (p. ej., hacer las tareas)	0	1	2	3

¿En qué medida los nueve comportamientos de la pregunta anterior le provocan problemas a su hijo/a?	Ningún problema	Problema menor	Problema moderado	Problema grave
Llevarse bien con familiars	0	1	2	3
Llevarse bien con otros niños	0	1	2	3
Completar o devolver las tareas escolares	0	1	2	3
Tener un buen desempeño académico en la escuela	0	1	2	3
Controlar su comportamiento en la escuela	0	1	2	3
Sentirse bien con él/ella mismo/a	0	1	2	3

|continued)

¿Con qué frecuencia su hijo/a tiene este comportamiento?	Nunca o rara vez	En ocasiones	A menudo	Con mucha frecuencia
Juguetea o golpea con las manos o los pies o se retuerce en el asiento	0	1	2	3
Se levanta en situaciones en que se espera que permanezca sentado/a	0	1	2	3
Corretea o trepa en situaciones en las que no resulta apropiado	0	1	2	3
Es incapaz de jugar o de ocuparse tranquilamente en actividades recreativas	0	1	2	3
Está "ocupado/a," actuando como si "lo impulsara un motor"	0	1	2	3
Habla excesivamente	0	1	2	3
Responde inesperadamente o antes de que se haya concluido una pregunta	0	1	2	3
Le es dificil esperar su turno (p. ej., mientras espera en una cola)	0	1	2	3
Interrumpe o se inmiscuye con otros	0	1	2	3

¿En qué medida los nueve comportamientos de la pregunta anterior le provocan problemas a su hijo/a?	Ningún problem	Problema menor	Problema moderado	Problema grave
Llevarse bien con familiares	0	1	2	3
Llevarse bien con otros niños	0	1	2	3
Completar o devolver las tareas escolares	0	1	2	3
Tener un buen desempeño académico en la escuela	0	1	2	3
Controlar su comportamiento en la escuela	0	1	2	3
Sentirse bien con él/ella mismo/a	0	1	2	3

Attention and Behavior Rating Form, Home Version: Adolescent (Spanish)

Edad del niño/niña: ______________________ Sexo: M F Grado: _____ País de origen: ____________

Completado por: Madre ____ Padre ____ Abuela/o ____ Otro parentesco ____

Seleccione la respuesta *que describe mejor el comportamiento de su hijo/a adolescente en los últimos 6 meses.*

¿Con qué frecuencia su hijo/a adolescente tiene este comportamiento?	Nunca o rara vez	En ocasiones	A menudo	Con mucha frecuencia
Falla en prestar la debida atención a detalles o por descuido se cometen errores en las tareas escolares, en el trabajo o durante otras actividades	0	1	2	3
Tiene dificultades para mantener la atención en tareas o actividades recreativas (p. ej., tiene dificultad para mantener la atención en conversaciones o la lectura prolongada)	0	1	2	3
Parece no escuchar cuando se le habla directamente	0	1	2	3
No sigue las instrucciones y no termina las tareas escolares, los quehaceres o los deberes laborales	0	1	2	3
Tiene dificultad para organizar tareas y actividades	0	1	2	3
Evita, le disgusta o se muestra poco entusiasta en iniciar tareas que requieren un esfuerzo mental sostenido (p. ej., tareas escolares o quehaceres domésticos; reparación de informes)	0	1	2	3
Pierde cosas necesarias para tareas o actividades (p. ej.,materiales escolares, lápices, libros, instrumentos, billetero, llaves, papeles del trabajo, gafas, móvil)	0	1	2	3
Se distrae con facilidad por estímulos externos	0	1	2	3
Olvida las actividades cotidianas (p. ej., hacer las tareas, hacer las diligencias, devolver las llamadas, acudir a las citas)	0	1	2	3

¿En qué medida los nueve comportamientos de la pregunta anterior le provocan problemas a su hijo/a adolescente?:	Ningún problema	Problema menor	Problema moderado	Problema grave
Llevarse bien con familiares	0	1	2	3
Llevarse bien con otros adolescents	0	1	2	3
Completar o devolver las tareas escolares	0	1	2	3
Tener un buen desempeño académico en la escuela	0	1	2	3
Controlar su comportamiento en la escuela	0	1	2	3
Sentirse bien con él/ella mismo/a	0	1	2	3

(continued)

¿Con qué frecuencia su hijo/a adolescente tiene este comportamiento?	Nunca o rara vez	En ocasiones	A menudo	Con mucha frecuencia
Juguetea o golpea con las manos o los pies o se retuerce en el asiento	0	1	2	3
Se levanta en situaciones en que se espera que permanezca sentado/a	0	1	2	3
Corretea o trepa en situaciones en las que no resulta apropiado o está inquieto	0	1	2	3
Es incapaz de jugar o de ocuparse tranquilamente en actividades recreativas	0	1	2	3
Está "ocupado/a," actuando como si "lo impulsara un motor" (p. ej., es incapaz de estar quieto/a o se siente incómodo/a estando quieto/a durante un tiempo prolongado)	0	1	2	3
Habla excesivamente	0	1	2	3
Responde inesperadamente o antes de que se haya concluido una pregunta	0	1	2	3
Le es dificil esperar su turno (p. ej., mientras espera en una cola)	0	1	2	3
Interrumpe o se inmiscuye con otros (p. ej., se mete en las conversaciones, juegos o actividades; peude inmiscuirse o adelantarse a lo que hacen otros)	0	1	2	3

¿En qué medida los nueve comportamientos de la pregunta anterior le provocan problemas a su hijo/a adolescente?:	Ningún problema	Problema menor	Problema moderado	Problema grave
Llevarse bien con familiares	0	1	2	3
Llevarse bien con otros adolescents	0	1	2	3
Completar o devolver las tareas escolares	0	1	2	3
Tener un buen desempeño académico en la escuela	0	1	2	3
Controlar su comportamiento en la escuela	0	1	2	3
Sentirse bien con él/ella mismo/a	0	1	2	3

ADHD Rating Scale–5, Home Version: Symptom Scoring Sheet for Boys

Child's name: ______________________ Date: __________ Age: __________

%ile	HI 5–7	HI 8–10	HI 11–13	HI 14–17	IA 5–7	IA 8–10	IA 11–13	IA 14–17	Total 5–7	Total 8–10	Total 11–13	Total 14–17	%ile
99+	27	27	26	21	27	27	27	27	50	53	52	47	99+
99	24	26	22	16	25	27	27	26	45	49	47	39	99
98	19	20	19	15	23	25	27	25	41	44	43	37	98
97	18	20	18	13	22	21	25	21	38	38	38	34	97
96	17	19	17	12	21	20	22	20	38	36	36	30	96
95	17	18	15	10	18	17	21	19	35	35	34	27	95
94	17	17	14	9	17	16	21	18	32	33	31	26	94
93	17	16	13	9	17	16	19	18	31	31	30	25	93
92	16	16	12	9	16	16	18	17	29	30	28	25	92
91	15	15	11	8	15	15	18	16	27	29	26	22	91
90	15	14	10	8	14	14	17	16	27	28	25	21	90
89	13	13	10	7	14	12	16	15	26	25	24	20	89
88	13	11	9	7	12	12	15	14	25	24	23	19	88
87	12	10	9	6	11	12	15	13	24	22	22	18	87
86	12	10	9	5	11	11	15	12	22	21	22	18	86
85	10	9	9	5	10	11	14	11	20	19	21	17	85
84	10	9	9	5	10	11	13	11	20	19	21	16	84
80	9	8	7	4	9	9	12	10	18	17	19	14	80
75	8	7	6	3	9	9	10	9	16	14	17	11	75
50	5	3	2	1	5	4	6	4	10	8	8	5	50
25	2	1	0	0	2	2	1	1	4	3	2	2	25
10	0	0	0	0	0	0	0	0	0	1	0	0	10
1	0	0	0	0	0	0	0	0	0	0	0	0	1

Note. HI, Hyperactivity–Impulsivity; IA, Inattention.

ADHD Rating Scale–5, Home Version: Symptom Scoring Sheet for Girls

Child's name: ______________________ Date: __________ Age: __________

%ile	HI 5–7	HI 8–10	HI 11–13	HI 14–17	IA 5–7	IA 8–10	IA 11–13	IA 14–17	Total 5–7	Total 8–10	Total 11–13	Total 14–17	%ile
99+	27	26	22	20	26	27	27	25	50	53	38	42	99+
99	25	23	16	19	23	26	25	23	45	47	35	36	99
98	20	21	15	12	21	22	21	19	43	37	32	32	98
97	17	15	14	11	18	18	20	18	35	36	29	28	97
96	16	13	13	9	17	17	19	18	32	30	29	25	96
95	15	11	12	9	16	16	17	18	29	28	27	24	95
94	14	10	12	8	15	15	15	17	27	25	24	23	94
93	13	9	11	8	14	14	15	17	25	21	23	21	93
92	12	9	9	7	13	13	13	15	24	21	22	20	92
91	12	9	9	6	13	13	13	14	22	20	21	20	91
90	11	9	8	6	12	12	12	14	21	20	20	19	90
89	10	8	8	6	12	12	12	13	21	18	19	18	89
88	9	8	7	5	12	11	11	13	20	18	18	18	88
87	9	8	7	5	12	11	11	12	18	17	18	17	87
86	8	7	7	5	11	11	10	12	18	17	18	16	86
85	8	7	6	4	10	10	10	11	18	16	17	15	85
84	8	7	6	4	10	10	10	11	17	16	16	15	84
80	7	6	5	3	9	9	9	9	15	14	13	12	80
75	6	5	4	3	8	8	8	7	13	12	11	10	75
50	3	2	1	1	3	3	3	3	7	6	5	4	50
25	1	0	0	0	1	1	1	0	3	2	1	1	25
10	0	0	0	0	0	0	0	0	0	0	0	0	10
1	0	0	0	0	0	0	0	0	0	0	0	0	1

Note. HI, Hyperactivity–Impulsivity; IA, Inattention.

ADHD Rating Scale–5, Home Version: Impairment Scoring Sheet for Boys

Child's name: ____________________ Date: __________ Age: __________

%ile	Family Relations				Peer Relations				Homework				Academics				Behavior				Self-Esteem				%ile
	5–7	8–10	11–13	14–17	5–7	8–10	11–13	14–17	5–7	8–10	11–13	14–17	5–7	8–10	11–13	14–17	5–7	8–10	11–13	14–17	5–7	8–10	11–13	14–17	
99.5+	3	3	3	3	3	3	3	3	3	3	3	3	3	3	3	3	3	3	3	3	3	3	2-3	3	99.5+
99			2				2	2		2										2		2		2	99
98	2	2		2	2	2					2			2				2	2		2				98
95				1				1	2			2	2		2	2	2			1	1			1	95
93		1	1		1	1	1							1								1	1		93
90	1								1	1			1					1	1						90
85											1	1			1	1	1								85
80								0																	80
75							0												0	0	0	0		0	75
70		0		0	0	0			0				0	0				0					0		70
65	0		0														0								65
60										0					0	0									60
55											0	0													55
50																									50

ADHD Rating Scale–5, Home Version: Impairment Scoring Sheet for Girls

Child's name: ______________________ Date: __________ Age: __________

	Family Relations				Peer Relations				Homework				Academics				Behavior				Self-Esteem				
%ile	5–7	8–10	11–13	14–17	5–7	8–10	11–13	14–17	5–7	8–10	11–13	14–17	5–7	8–10	11–13	14–17	5–7	8–10	11–13	14–17	5–7	8–10	11–13	14–17	%ile
99.5+	3	3	3	3	2-3	3	3	3	2-3	3	3	3	3	3	3	3	3	2-3	3	3	2-3	2-3	3	3	99.5+
99	2	2	2			2	2			2			2				2		2						99
98					1			2			2	2		2	2	2		1		2	1		2	2	98
95	1	1		2		1	1		1	1			1	1			1		1	1		1			95
93															1								1	1	93
90			1					1			1	1													90
85				1									0			1				0	0				85
80					0				0									0	0						80
75						0	0			0	0			0	0		0					0			75
70	0	0						0															0		70
65			0													0								0	65
60				0								0													60
55																									55
50																									50

Attention and Behavior Rating Form, School Version: Child

Student's name: ____________________ Sex: M F Age: ______ Grade: ________________

Completed by: ____

Please select the answer that *best describes this student's behavior over the past 6 months (or since the beginning of the school year).*

How often does this child display this behavior?	Never or Rarely	Sometimes	Often	Very Often
Fails to give close attention to details or makes careless mistakes in schoolwork or during other activities	0	1	2	3
Has difficulty sustaining attention in tasks or play activities	0	1	2	3
Does not seem to listen when spoken to directly	0	1	2	3
Does not follow through on instructions and fails to finish schoolwork	0	1	2	3
Has difficulty organizing tasks and activities	0	1	2	3
Avoids, dislikes, or is reluctant to engage in tasks that require sustained mental effort (e.g., schoolwork or homework)	0	1	2	3
Loses things necessary for tasks or activities (e.g., school materials, pencils, books)	0	1	2	3
Easily distracted by extraneous stimuli	0	1	2	3
Forgetful in daily activities	0	1	2	3

How much do the nine behaviors in the previous question cause problems for this child?	No Problem	Minor Problem	Moderate Problem	Severe Problem
Getting along with school professionals	0	1	2	3
Getting along with other children	0	1	2	3
Completing or returning homework	0	1	2	3
Performing academically in school	0	1	2	3
Controlling behavior in school	0	1	2	3
Feeling good about himself/herself	0	1	2	3

(continued)

Attention and Behavior Rating Form, School Version: Child *(page 2 of 2)*

How often does this child display this behavior?	Never or Rarely	Sometimes	Often	Very Often
Fidgets with or taps hands or feet or squirms in seat	0	1	2	3
Leaves seat in situations when remaining seated is expected	0	1	2	3
Runs about or climbs in situations where it is inappropriate	0	1	2	3
Unable to play or engage in leisure activities quietly	0	1	2	3
"On the go," acts as if "driven by a motor"	0	1	2	3
Talks excessively	0	1	2	3
Blurts out an answer before a question has been completed	0	1	2	3
Has difficulty waiting his or her turn (e.g., while waiting in line).	0	1	2	3
Interrupts or intrudes on others	0	1	2	3

How much do the nine behaviors in the previous question cause problems for this child?	No Problem	Minor Problem	Moderate Problem	Severe Problem
Getting along with school professionals	0	1	2	3
Getting along with other children	0	1	2	3
Completing or returning homework	0	1	2	3
Performing academically in school	0	1	2	3
Controlling behavior in school	0	1	2	3
Feeling good about himself/herself	0	1	2	3

Attention and Behavior Rating Form, School Version: Adolescent

Student's name: ______________________ Sex: M F Age: _______ Grade: _______________

Completed by: ____

Please select the answer that *best describes this student's behavior over the past 6 months (or since the beginning of the school year).*

How often does this student display this behavior?	Never or Rarely	Sometimes	Often	Very Often
Fails to give close attention to details or makes careless mistakes in schoolwork or during other activities	0	1	2	3
Has difficulty sustaining attention in tasks or play activities (e.g., has difficulty remaining focused during lectures, conversations or lengthy reading)	0	1	2	3
Does not seem to listen when spoken to directly	0	1	2	3
Does not follow through on instructions and fails to finish schoolwork	0	1	2	3
Has difficulty organizing tasks and activities	0	1	2	3
Avoids, dislikes, or is reluctant to engage in tasks that require sustained mental effort (e.g., schoolwork or homework; preparing reports)	0	1	2	3
Loses things necessary for tasks or activities (e.g., school materials, pencils, books)	0	1	2	3
Easily distracted by extraneous stimuli or unrelated thoughts	0	1	2	3
Forgetful in daily activities	0	1	2	3

How much do the nine behaviors in the previous question cause problems for this student?	No Problem	Minor Problem	Moderate Problem	Severe Problem
Getting along with school professionals	0	1	2	3
Getting along with other students	0	1	2	3
Completing or returning homework	0	1	2	3
Performing academically in school	0	1	2	3
Controlling behavior in school	0	1	2	3
Feeling good about himself/herself	0	1	2	3

(continued)

How often does this student display this behavior?	Never or Rarely	Sometimes	Often	Very Often
Fidgets with or taps hands or feet or squirms in seat	0	1	2	3
Leaves seat in situations when remaining seated is expected	0	1	2	3
Runs about or climbs in situations where it is inappropriate or feels restless	0	1	2	3
Unable to play or engage in leisure activities quietly	0	1	2	3
"On the go," acts as if "driven by a motor" (e.g., unable to be or uncomfortable being still for an extended time)	0	1	2	3
Talks excessively	0	1	2	3
Blurts out an answer before a question has been completed	0	1	2	3
Has difficulty waiting his or her turn (e.g., while waiting in line).	0	1	2	3
Interrupts or intrudes on others (e.g., butts into conversations, games, or activities; may intrude into or take over what others are doing)	0	1	2	3

How much do the nine behaviors in the previous question cause problems for this student?	No Problem	Minor Problem	Moderate Problem	Severe Problem
Getting along with school professionals	0	1	2	3
Getting along with other students	0	1	2	3
Completing or returning homework	0	1	2	3
Performing academically in school	0	1	2	3
Controlling behavior in school	0	1	2	3
Feeling good about himself/herself	0	1	2	3

ADHD Rating Scale–5, School Version: Symptom Scoring Sheet for Boys

Student's name: ______________________ Date: __________ Age: __________

%ile	HI 5–7	HI 8–10	HI 11–13	HI 14–17	IA 5–7	IA 8–10	IA 11–13	IA 14–17	Total 5–7	Total 8–10	Total 11–13	Total 14–17	%ile
99+	27	27	26	27	27	27	27	27	50	54	52	54	99+
99	27	27	24	26	27	27	27	27	50	54	50	53	99
98	26	26	23	23	27	27	27	27	48	50	46	44	98
97	25	23	22	19	26	27	26	24	45	48	45	39	97
96	24	22	21	17	25	26	25	22	43	44	41	37	96
95	23	22	19	16	25	26	25	21	42	44	39	35	95
94	21	21	19	14	24	24	25	21	42	42	38	32	94
93	20	20	18	14	22	24	24	20	40	40	38	31	93
92	19	19	18	13	22	24	24	20	39	39	37	30	92
91	18	19	17	13	21	23	23	19	38	38	36	29	91
90	18	18	16	12	20	22	23	18	38	36	35	27	90
89	18	17	15	12	20	22	22	17	37	36	33	26	89
88	18	17	15	11	20	20	21	16	36	35	33	25	88
87	17	16	14	11	20	19	21	16	35	35	32	25	87
86	17	16	14	10	18	19	20	15	34	34	32	25	86
85	17	16	13	10	18	19	20	15	33	33	31	24	85
84	17	15	13	10	18	18	19	15	32	32	30	23	84
80	14	14	10	8	17	18	18	13	30	30	29	20	80
75	13	12	9	6	14	16	15	12	26	27	25	18	75
50	6	5	3	1	9	9	8	6	14	15	12	8	50
25	1	0	0	0	2	2	2	1	5	3	3	2	25
10	0	0	0	0	0	0	0	0	1	0	0	0	10
1	0	0	0	0	0	0	0	0	0	0	0	0	1

Note. HI, Hyperactivity–Impulsivity; IA, Inattention.

ADHD Rating Scale–5, School Version: Symptom Scoring Sheet for Girls

Student's name: ______________________ Date: __________ Age: __________

%ile	HI 5–7	HI 8–10	HI 11–13	HI 14–17	IA 5–7	IA 8–10	IA 11–13	IA 14–17	Total 5–7	Total 8–10	Total 11–13	Total 14–17	%ile
99+	24	23	27	26	24	27	27	27	45	48	53	52	99+
99	24	20	23	21	24	26	26	27	45	41	46	46	99
98	21	18	18	15	23	24	25	25	43	40	41	33	98
97	20	18	15	13	23	23	24	20	42	37	38	31	97
96	19	15	13	12	22	21	23	18	38	35	33	29	96
95	17	15	13	10	20	20	22	16	36	33	31	25	95
94	16	15	12	9	19	19	22	15	33	31	30	23	94
93	15	14	11	9	18	19	21	14	33	31	29	22	93
92	15	13	11	9	18	18	20	14	31	30	28	21	92
91	14	13	10	8	17	18	19	13	30	29	27	20	91
90	14	13	9	7	17	18	18	12	30	28	26	19	90
89	14	11	9	6	17	17	17	11	29	27	25	18	89
88	14	11	9	6	16	17	16	11	29	25	25	16	88
87	14	10	9	5	16	17	16	11	28	24	23	16	87
86	13	10	9	5	16	16	15	10	27	24	22	14	86
85	12	9	8	5	15	15	14	10	26	23	22	14	85
84	11	9	8	5	15	15	14	9	26	22	21	14	84
80	9	7	6	3	13	12	12	8	22	20	18	11	80
75	8	6	4	2	11	11	10	7	18	17	15	9	75
50	2	2	1	0	3	5	3	2	6	7	5	3	50
25	0	0	0	0	0	0	0	0	1	1	1	0	25
10	0	0	0	0	0	0	0	0	0	0	0	0	10
1	0	0	0	0	0	0	0	0	0	0	0	0	1

Note. HI, Hyperactivity–Impulsivity; IA, Inattention.

ADHD Rating Scale–5, School Version: Impairment Scoring Sheet for Boys

Student's name: ______________________ Date: __________ Age: __________

	Teacher Relations				Peer Relations				Homework				Academics				Behavior				Self-Esteem				
%ile	5–7	8–10	11–13	14–17	5–7	8–10	11–13	14–17	5–7	8–10	11–13	14–17	5–7	8–10	11–13	14–17	5–7	8–10	11–13	14–17	5–7	8–10	11–13	14–17	%ile
99.5+	3	3	3	3	3	3	3	3	3	3	3	3	3	3	3	3	3	3	3	3	3	3	3	3	99.5+
99																									99
98	2	2	2	2	2		2	2													2		2	2	98
95						2													2	2		2			95
93																									93
90								1	2		2	2	2		2	2	2	2						1	90
85	1	1	1	1			1			2													1		85
80					1	1								2					1	1	1	1			80
75									1																75
70										1	1	1	1		1	1	1							0	70
65			0	0				0																	65
60	0						0							1				1					0		60
55		0																		0		0			55
50						0													0		0				50
45					0				0	0					0										45
40											0	0	0	0		0	0	0							40

ADHD Rating Scale–5, School Version: Impairment Scoring Sheet for Girls

Student's name: ______________________ Date: __________ Age: __________

	Teacher Relations				Peer Relations				Homework				Academics				Behavior				Self-Esteem				
%ile	5–7	8–10	11–13	14–17	5–7	8–10	11–13	14–17	5–7	8–10	11–13	14–17	5–7	8–10	11–13	14–17	5–7	8–10	11–13	14–17	5–7	8–10	11–13	14–17	**%ile**
99.5+	2–3	3	3	3	3	3	3	3	3	3	3	3	3	3	3	3	3	3	3	3	3	3	3	3	99.5+
99		2		2		2		2															2	2	99
98			2		2		2	1	2			2				2			2	2		2			98
95										2							2	2			2				95
93	1	1	1	1										2						1			1	1	93
90						1	1				2	1	2		2				1			1			90
85					1											1		1		0	1				85
80				0				0	1	1	1		1												80
75	0	0	0				0							1	1		1							0	75
70																			0		0		0		70
65												0				0		0				0			65
60					0	0				0															60
55									0				0	0	0		0								55
50											0														50
45																									45
40																									40

References

Achenbach, T. M. (1991a). *Integrative guide for the 1991 CBCL/4–18, YSR, and TRF Profiles*. Burlington: University of Vermont, Department of Psychiatry.

Achenbach, T. M. (1991b). *Manual for the Child Behavior Checklist/4–18 and 1991 Profile*. Burlington: University of Vermont, Department of Psychiatry.

Achenbach, T. M. (1991c). *Manual for the Teacher's Report Form and 1991 Profile*. Burlington: University of Vermont, Department of Psychiatry.

American Psychiatric Association. (1968). *Diagnostic and statistical manual of mental disorders* (2nd ed.). Washington, DC: Author.

American Psychiatric Association. (1980). *Diagnostic and statistical manual of mental disorders* (3rd ed.). Washington, DC: Author.

American Psychiatric Association. (1987). *Diagnostic and statistical manual of mental disorders* (3rd ed., rev.). Washington, DC: Author.

American Psychiatric Association. (2013). *Diagnostic and statistical manual of mental disorders* (5th ed.). Arlington, VA: Author.

American Psychiatric Association. (2014). *Guía de consulta de los criterios diagnósticos del DSM-5*. Arlington, VA: Author.

Anastopoulos, A. D., & Shelton, T. L. (2011). Assessing treatment response. In S. W. Evans & B. Hoza (Eds.), *Treating attention deficit hyperactivity disorder* (pp. 7.1–7.19). Kingston, NJ: Civic Research Institute.

Barkley, R. A. (1990). *Attention-deficit hyperactivity disorder: A handbook for diagnosis and treatment*. New York: Guilford Press.

Barkley, R. A. (Ed.). (2015). *Attention-deficit/hyperactivity disorder: A handbook for diagnosis and treatment* (4th ed.). New York: Guilford Press.

Bauermeister, J. J., Bird, H. R., Canino, G., Rubio-Stipec, M., Bravo, M., & Alegria, M. (1995). Dimensions of attention deficit hyperactivity disorder: Findings from teacher and parent reports in a community sample. *Journal of Clinical Child Psychology, 24*, 264–271.

Bentler, P. M. (1990). Comparative fit indexes in structural models. *Psychological Bulletin, 107*, 238–246.

Boomsma, A. (2000). Reporting analyses of covariance structures. *Structural Equation Modeling, 7*, 461–483.

Browne, M. W., & Cudeck, R. (1993). Alternative ways of assessing model fit. In K. A. Bollen & J. S. Long (Eds.), *Testing structure equation models* (pp. 136–162). London: Sage.

Burns, G. L., Boe, B., Walsh, J. A., Sommers-Flanagan, R., & Teegarden, L. A. (2001). A confirmatory factor analysis on the DSM-IV ADHD and ODD symptoms: What is the best model for the organization of these symptoms? *Journal of Abnormal Child Psychology, 29*, 339–349.

Cauce, A. M., Domenech-Rodríguez, M., Paradise, M., Cochran, B. N., Shea, J. M., Srebnik, D., et al. (2002). Cultural and contextual influences in mental health help-seeking: A focus on ethnic minority youth. *Journal of Consulting and Clinical Psychology, 70*, 44–55.

Chen, W. J., Faraone, S. V., Biederman, J., & Tsuang, M. T. (1994). Diagnostic accuracy of the Child Behavior Checklist Scales for attention-deficit hyperactivity disorder: A receiver operating characteristic analysis. *Journal of Consulting and Clinical Psychology, 62*, 1017–1025.

Cheung, G. W., & Rensvold, R. B. (2002). Evaluating goodness-of-fit indexes for testing measurement invariance. *Structural Equation Modeling, 9*, 233–255.

Conners, C. K. (2008). *Conners 3rd edition*. Toronto: Multi-Health Systems.

DeMaris, A. (2013). Logistic regression: Basic foundations and new directions. In I. B. Weiner, J. A. Schinka, & W. F. Velicer (Eds.), *Handbook of psychology: Research methods in psychology* (2nd ed., Vol. 2, pp. 543–570). Hoboken, NJ: Wiley.

deRamirez, R. D., & Shapiro, E. S. (2005). Effects of student ethnicity on judgments of ADHD among Hispanic and white teachers. *School Psychology Quarterly, 20*, 268–287.

DiStefano, C., & Morgan, G. B. (2014). A comparison of diagonal weighted least square: A robust estimation technique for ordinal data. *Structural Equation Modeling, 21*, 425–438.

DuPaul, G. J., Anastopoulos, A. D., Power, T. J., Reid, R., Ikeda, M., & McGoey, K. (1998). Parent ratings of attention-deficit/hyperactivity disorder symptoms: Factor structure and normative data. *Journal of Psychopathology and Behavioral Assessment, 20*, 83–102.

DuPaul, G. J., Power, T. J., Anastopoulos, A. D., & Reid, R. (1998). *ADHD Rating Scale–IV: Checklists, norms, and clinical interpretation*. New York: Guilford Press.

DuPaul, G. J., Power, T. J., Anastopoulos, A. D., Reid, R., McGoey, K., & Ikeda, M. (1997). Teacher ratings of attention-deficit/hyperactivity disorder: Factor structure and normative data. *Psychological Assessment, 9*, 436–444.

DuPaul, G. J., Power, T. J., McGoey, K., Ikeda, M., & Anastopoulos, A. D. (1998). Reliability and validity of parent and teacher ratings of attention-deficit/hyperactivity disorder symptoms. *Journal of Psychoeducational Assessment, 16*, 55–68.

DuPaul, G. J., Reid, R., Anastopoulos, A. D., Lambert, M. C., Watkins, M. W., & Power, T. J. (2015, May 25). Parent and teacher ratings of attention-deficit/hyperactivity disorder symptoms: Factor structure and normative data. *Psychological Assessment*. Advance online publication. Available at *http://dx.doi.org/10.1037/pas0000166*.

DuPaul, G. J., Reid, R., Anastopoulos, A. D., & Power, T. J. (2014). Assessing ADHD symptomatic behaviors and functional impairment in school settings: Impact of student and teacher characteristics. *School Psychology Quarterly, 29*, 409–421.

DuPaul, G. J., & Stoner, G. (2014). *ADHD in the schools: Assessment and intervention strategies* (3rd ed.). New York: Guilford Press.

Eiraldi, R., Mazzuca, L., Clarke, A., & Power, T. (2006). Service utilization among ethnic minority children with ADHD: A model of help-seeking behavior. *Administration and Policy in Mental Health and Mental Health Services Research, 33*, 607–622.

Eiraldi, R. B., Power, T. J., & Nezu, C. M. (1997). Patterns of comorbidity associated with subtypes of attention-deficit/hyperactivity disorder among 6–12-year-old children. *Journal of the American Academy of Child and Adolescent Psychiatry, 36*, 503–514.

Epstein, J. N., Willoughby, M., Valencia, E. Y., Tonev, S. T., Abikoff, H. B., Arnold, L. E., et al. (2005). The role of children's ethnicity in the relationship between teacher ratings of attention-deficit/hyperactivity disorder and observed classroom behavior. *Journal of Consulting and Clinical Psychology, 73*, 424–434.

Evans, S. W., Brady, C. E., Harrison, J. R., Bunford, N., Kern, L., State, T., et al. (2013). Measuring ADHD and ODD symptoms and impairment using high school teachers' ratings. *Journal of Clinical Child and Adolescent Psychology, 42*, 197–207.

Fabiano, G. A., Pelham, W. E., Jr., Waschbusch, D. A., Gnagy, E. M., Lahey, B. B., Chronis, A. M., et al. (2006). A practical measure of impairment: Psychometric properties of the impairment rating scale in samples of children with attention deficit hyperactivity disorder and two school-based samples. *Journal of Clinical Child and Adolescent Psychology, 35*, 369–385.

Frick, P. J., Lahey, B. B., Applegate, B., Kerdyck, L., Ollendick, T., Hynd, G. W., et al. (1994). DSM-IV field trials for the disruptive behavior disorders: Symptom utility estimates. *Journal of the American Academy of Child and Adolescent Psychiatry, 33*, 529–539.

Fryer, R. G., & Levitt, S. D. (2004). Understanding the black-white test score gap in the first two years of school. *Review of Economics and Statistics, 86*, 447–464.

Garson, G. D. (2014). *Logistic regression: Binary and multinomial.* Asheboro, NC: Statistical Publishing Associates.

Gorsuch, R. L. (1997). Exploratory factor analysis: Its role in item analysis. *Journal of Personality Assessment, 68*, 532–560.

Hollingshead, A. B. (1975). *Four factor index of social status.* New Haven, CT: Yale University Press.

Hu, L., & Bentler, P. M. (1999). Cutoff criteria for fit indexes in covariance structure analysis: Conventional criteria versus new alternatives. *Structural Equation Modeling, 6*, 1–55.

Jacobsen, N. S., & Truax, P. (1991). Clinical significance: A statistical approach to defining meaningful change in psychotherapy research. *Journal of Consulting and Clinical Psychology, 59*, 12–19.

Karpenko, V., Owens, J. S., Evangelista, N. M., & Dodds, C. (2009). Clinically significant symptom change in children with attention-deficit/hyperactivity disorder: Does it correspond with reliable improvement in functioning? *Journal of Clinical Psychology, 65*(1), 76–93.

Kaufman, A. S., & Kaufman, N. L. (1990). *Kaufman Brief Intelligence Test.* Circle Pines, MN: American Guidance Service.

Langberg, J. M., Molina, B. S. G., Arnold, L. E., Epstein, J. N., Altaye, M., Hinshaw, S. P., et al. (2011). Patterns and predictors of adolescent academic achievement and performance in a sample of children with attention-deficit/hyperactivity disorder (ADHD). *Journal of Clinical Child and Adolescent Psychology, 40*(4), 519–531.

Laurent, J., Landau, S., & Stark, K. D. (1993). Conditional probabilities in the diagnosis of depressive and anxiety disorders in children. *School Psychology Review, 22*, 98–114.

Muthén, L. K., & Muthén, B. O. (1998–2014). *Mplus user's guide* (7th ed.). Los Angeles: Muthén & Muthén.

Nigg, J. T. (2001). Is ADHD a disinhibitory disorder? *Psychological Bulletin, 127*, 571–598.

Owens, J. S., Johannes, L. M., & Karpenko, V. (2009). The relation between change in symptoms and functioning in children with ADHD receiving school-based mental health services. *School Mental Health, 1*(4), 183–195.

Petrucci, C. J. (2009). A primer for social worker researchers on how to conduct a multinomial logistic regression. *Journal of Social Service Research, 35*, 193–205.

Polanczyk, G., de Lima, M. S., Horta, B. L., Biederman, J., & Rohde, L. A. (2007). The worldwide prevalence of ADHD: A systematic review and metaregression analysis. *American Journal of Psychiatry, 164*, 942–948.

Power, T. J., Andrews, T. J., Eiraldi, R. B., Doherty, B. J., Ikeda, M. J., DuPaul, G. J., et al. (1998). Evaluating attention deficit hyperactivity disorder using multiple informants: The incremental utility of combining teacher with parent reports. *Psychological Assessment, 10*, 250–260.

Power, T. J., & Bradley-Klug, K. L. (2013). *Pediatric school psychology: Conceptualization, applications, and strategies for leadership development.* New York: Routledge/Taylor & Francis.

Power, T. J., Doherty, B. J., Panichelli-Mindel, S. M., Karustis, J. L., Eiraldi, R. B., Anastopoulos, A. D., et al. (1998). The predictive validity of parent and teacher reports of ADHD symptoms. *Journal of Psychopathology and Behavioral Assessment, 20*, 57–81.

Power, T. J., Watkins, M. W., Anastopoulos, A. D., Reid, R., Lambert, M. C., & DuPaul, G. J. (2015). Multi-informant assessment of ADHD symptom-related impairments among children and adolescents. *Journal of Clinical Child and Adolescent Psychology.* Advance online publication.

Power, T. J., Werba, B. E., Watkins, M. W., Angelucci, J. G., & Eiraldi, R. B. (2006). Patterns of parent-reported homework problems among ADHD-referred and non-referred children. *School Psychology Quarterly, 21*(1), 13–33.

Reich, W., Shayka, M. A., & Taibleson, C. (1991). *Diagnostic Interview for Children and Adolescents–DSM-III-R Version (Parent Form).* St. Louis, MO: Washington University Division of Child Psychiatry.

Reid, R., DuPaul, G. J., Power, T. J., Anastopoulos, A. D., Rodgers-Adkinson, D., Noll, M. B., et al. (1998). Assessing culturally different students for attention-deficit/hyperactivity disorder using behavior rating scales. *Journal of Abnormal Child Psychology, 26*, 187–198.

Reynolds, R. C., & Kamphaus, W. R. (2004). *Behavior Assessment System for Children manual* (2nd ed.). Circle Pines, MN: AGS Publishing.

Shapiro, E. S. (2011). *Academic skills problems fourth edition workbook*. New York: Guilford Press.

Shemmassian, S. K., & Lee, S. S. (2012). Comparing four methods of integrating parent and teacher symptom ratings of attention-deficit/hyperactivity disorder (ADHD). *Journal of Psychopathology and Behavioral Assessment, 34*, 1–10.

Steiger, J. H., & Lind, J. C. (1980, May). *Statistically-based tests for the number of common factors*. Paper presented at the annual spring meeting of the Psychometric Society, Iowa City, IA.

Ullebø, A. K., Breivik, K., Gillberg, C., Lundervold, A. J., & Posserud, M. B. (2012). The factor structure of ADHD in a general population of primary school children. *Journal of Child Psychology and Psychiatry, 53*, 927–936.

Verhulst, F. C., & Koot, H. M. (1992). *Child psychiatric epidemiology: Concepts, methods, and findings*. Newbury Park, CA: Sage.

Visser, S. N., Danielson, M. L., Bitsko, R. H., Holbrook, J. R., Kogan, M. D., Ghandour, R. M., et al. (2014). Trends in the parent-report of health care provider-diagnosed and medicated attention-deficit/hyperactivity disorder: United States, 2003–2011. *Journal of the American Academy of Child and Adolescent Psychiatry, 53*, 34–46.

Wainer, H. (1976). Estimating coefficients in linear models: It don't make no nevermind. *Psychological Bulletin, 83*, 213–217.

Willcutt, E. G. (2012). The prevalence of DSM-IV attention-deficit/hyperactivity disorder: A meta-analytic review. *Neurotherapeutics, 9*, 490–499.

Index

Page numbers followed by *f* indicate figure, *t* indicate table

B

C

D

E

R

S

T

V